Waistland

Also by Deirdre Barrett

Trauma and Dreams

*The Pregnant Man
and Other Cases from a Hypnotherapist's Couch*

The Committee of Sleep

The New Science of Dreaming

Waistland

The (R)Evolutionary Science

behind Our Weight

and Fitness Crisis

Deirdre Barrett

W · W · Norton & Company

New York • London

For information about permission to reproduce selections from this book,
write to Permissions, W. W. Norton & Company, Inc.,
500 Fifth Avenue, New York, NY 10110

For information about special discounts for bulk purchases,
please contact W. W. Norton Special Sales at
specialsales@wwnorton.com or 800-233-4830

Manufacturing by R.R. Donnelley
Book design by Margaret M. Wagner
Production manager: Julia Druskin

Library of Congress Cataloging-in-Publication Data

Barrett, Deirdre.
Waistland : the (R)evolutionary science behind our weight and fitness
crisis / Deirdre Barrett. — 1st ed.
p. cm.
Includes bibliographical references and index.
ISBN 978-0-393-06216-8 (hardcover)
1. Obesity — United States. 2. Food habits. 3. Weight loss. 4. Human
evolution. 5. Physical fitness. I. Title.
RA645.O2337 2007
613.7'12 — dc22

2007011136

W. W. Norton & Company, Inc.
500 Fifth Avenue, New York, N.Y. 10110
www.wwnorton.com

W. W. Norton & Company Ltd.
Castle House, 75/76 Wells Street, W1T 3QT

1 2 3 4 5 6 7 8 9 0

Contents

Waistland

1

Don't Feed the Animals

Zoos across America post signs: "DON'T FEED THE ANIMALS." To young children, this looks mean-spirited. If they love the cute otter turning flips, why not share their potato chips or marshmallow cups? Adults quickly explain that what animals need is meat, fish, greens or chow pellets carefully engineered for a balance of nutrients. This is otter meal . . . lion food . . . elephant chow. The children's well-intentioned offerings would make the animals fat, sick, short-lived. Chips and candy are *human food.*

What's wrong with this picture?

We're similarly perverse when it comes to exercise. People rarely keep a dog in the city unless there's a yard or park nearby. A wheel is minimum equipment for a hamster cage—many now have elaborate gyms or mazes. We know pets grow unhappy and unhealthy without exercise. But how many people spend hours in front of a television without even thinking of getting on a treadmill or stair-climber (remarkably like modern, human hamster wheels), much less going for a run?

Years ago, zoo animals confined in small cages lay around,

3

fought or bit their own skin. They behaved like people suffering from depression and neurosis. Zookeepers noticed and responded, and now you see animals in larger, more natural enclosures. When are we going to start being humane to humans—why don't we make the same connection about how much of our rising rate of depression is due to inactivity? We're raising free-range chickens to feed to couch-potato people.

—

By 1995, America's government, press and public were desperately aware that we were in the grip of an epidemic of enormous proportions—literally. Two-thirds of Americans were overweight. Obesity was killing 300,000 people a year, sickening millions and costing $99 billion annually in medical costs. Weight-related illnesses were poised to overtake smoking as the major preventable cause of death.[1] Excess weight was the single most common thing people said they disliked about their own bodies. Two-thirds of Americans ranked losing weight as a goal of moderate to high importance.[2]

So what changes have we made in the intervening decade? We've eaten 50 percent more fast-food meals and five more pounds of sugar a year. We've increased the number of vending machines in our schools and decreased physical education programs.[3] US obesity-related health costs have risen to $117 billion[4] and medical epidemiologists now estimate that eight out of ten Americans will eventually become overweight.[5] Fewer Americans are dieting than a decade ago—and with less success.[6] In 2004, the World Health Organization proposed dietary guidelines to reduce fat and sugar consumption. The US delegation—representing the fattest nation in the world—protested this, on behalf of the food industry, as "scientifically unproven."[7]

What's going on?

We know we have a weight problem but we're still looking

for an easy way out—and many diet programs encourage such fantasies. There are some diet myths that everyone now knows are false, even if we're tempted to hang onto them as excuses:

- You can diet to lose weight, then go back to eating as usual
- You only need to eat heart-healthy after a heart attack
- "Home-baked" must be good for you

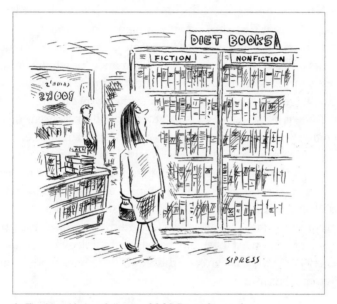

(© The New Yorker Collection 2002 David Sipress from cartoonbank.com)

But there's a new set of diet myths:

- It doesn't matter if you slip once in a while
- A food "treat" is a good way to reinforce a diet
- Diets shouldn't be too extreme or you won't stick with them
- To stop overeating, you should "listen to your body"

- The ideal you see in actresses and "Miss America" is too thin for health; this "unrealistic" ideal is fueling the obesity epidemic

Not one of these is true.

Slips from a diet or treats to reinforce one unleash a cascade of biochemical events: glucose, insulin and at least three different "hunger hormones" all shoot upward. It's much harder to stick with your diet the day after a lapse. I'm going to tell you not to listen to your body—at least not to its inborn preferences for fats and sugar or its conditioned demands for whatever junk foods you've eaten recently. And I'm going to tell you that radical changes are necessary. Small ones just won't do it.

There is a "good news" side to this. At first, swearing off French fries sounds harder than ordering the small size, more difficult than a regimen where weight loss is rewarded with a serving of your favorite dessert. But research shows that in terms of habits and substances, radical changes are often *easier*. If it's a hardship to go a week without eating a single cookie, then it's natural to assume that it would feel infinitely worse to go five years without one. However, the basic physiology of substance addiction means that after withdrawal, hormones readjust and cravings diminish.

The first chapters of this book will describe what kind of diet our bodies are actually designed for and how modern menus have subverted our instincts to make us overeat. I'll challenge the myth that our current ideal is either too thin or much thinner than in most past eras.

The later chapters will describe what we—as individuals and as a society—need to do to reverse this deadly trend. I draw on my years as a therapist and faculty member at Harvard's Behavioral Medicine Program for the most effective ways to lose weight: imagery and cognitive-behavioral restructuring. These techniques teach people to *listen to logic* and to eat foods that dampen rather than fuel hunger. I'll describe some of my patients and others who have beaten the evolutionary odds to lose weight and keep it off despite modern society's unprecedented challenges.

Our government, like us, has been hoping for an easy way out, pretending vague dietary guidelines will reverse the obesity epidemic and avoiding confrontations with America's powerful food lobby. There's an upside here, too: farmers can make at least the same money from broccoli if the government switches from subsidizing the growing of corn syrup to subsidizing the growing of healthy vegetables. I'll describe the radical changes necessary in advertising laws and food subsidies if we—as a society rather than as a few maverick individuals—are going to get healthy.

Waistland will argue that we must view the basic problem from the vantage point of evolution. A recurring concept throughout the book will be that of "supernormal stimuli." This term, borrowed from ethology (the study of animal behavior), refers to artificial objects that appeal to our instincts *more* than the natural foods or activities for which those instincts were designed. We're programmed to forage for sugar and saturated fats because these were once found only in hard-to-come-by fruit and game. Now this programming lures us powerfully toward plastic-wrapped hunks of corn syrup solids and hydrogenated vegetable oils. Similarly hijacked instincts make us sit immobile for hours in front of electronic displays of other people's lives. We're hunter-gatherers lost in a jungle of burgers, lounge chairs and TV remotes.

This book doesn't present a new diet—that's the last thing we need. It does challenge a few diet truisms that are actually very bad advice. But most diet and fitness recommendations are sound and *simple*—get more exercise, eat fewer calories, get those calories from vegetables and fish. Polls show that 95 percent of

Americans know this, yet only 5 percent follow it. We'll examine smoking cessation as an analogous problem that was recognized decades before society got serious about reversing the trend. We'll explore evolutionary perspectives that help explain *why* people aren't following the recommendations, what's wrong with current approaches to fitness and what *will* work—both for the individual and for society.

People were concerned with weight and overeating long before obesity rose to its current epidemic level. To find the origin of the problem, we need to go far back in time. The next chapter will explore prehistoric eras and see what the fossil evidence suggests about when obesity and associated health problems began to appear.

2

Which Came First: the Take-Out Fried Chicken or the Cholesterol-Laden Egg?

> The greater part of our ills are of our own making and we might have avoided them nearly all, by adhering to the simple . . . manner of life which nature prescribed . . . In following the history of civil society we shall be telling that of human sickness.
>
> —JEAN-JACQUES ROUSSEAU, *1754*

To plan effective diet and fitness strategies, we need to understand human evolution. Before we "listen to the body," we must know the environment for which it's programmed. This basic idea is often ignored, and people expect to have correct instincts about how to respond to modern foods.

In some vicious cycles, we don't know which component came first. With the evolution of our current obesity epidemic, we do. It is tempting to blame fast-food chains and self-interested advertisers for creating our desire for fats, sugar and salt, but this is not the case. They play on them, compound them, profit from them—but they did not create them. The "egg" half of the

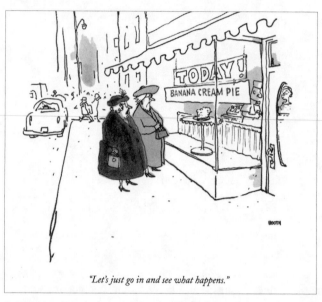

"Let's just go in and see what happens."

cycle—our craving for the fat in egg yolks—preceded the "fried chicken" half—foods and advertising developed to cater to that desire for fat. If we started out hard wired for small portions over large or soy over bologna, advertisers would happily reinforce these preferences instead—they'd be even cheaper to supply. In Chapter 3, we'll explore the "fried chicken" half of the cycle and how marketing does contribute to the problem. First, however, we'll examine the "egg" half, to understand the setting in which humans evolved and its impact on our food cravings today.

The Good Old Days: 8000 BC

The average person might think back fifty to seventy years for a model of "natural" food: the classic American farm of our grandparents' era. But that farm already had a fried chicken recipe . . . and the early signs of our obesity/unfitness epidemic. The US government has kept records on military recruits for more than 150 years, and the average weight for height has increased steadily from their earliest measurements.[1] Evolutionary anthropologists look back more than ten thousand years to understand our natural lifestyle and diet.

Ten thousand years is how long humans have been farming. That may sound like a long time, but it equals only 1 percent of human history. The genes regulating enzymes to digest food and convert it into healthy tissue and energy were shaped over thousands of generations and over hundreds of thousands of years.

Until about 8000 BC, all humans lived as hunter-gatherers. They depended on wild foods: hunting, fishing and trapping small animals, and gathering fruits, tubers, leaves and seeds. They consumed most foods within days—usually hours—of obtaining them. Gathering activities temporarily depleted the local food supply, so they moved their camps every few days or months.

A generation ago, it was popular to refer to this lifestyle as "primitive." The Stone Age was pictured as a time of fear, toil and danger in which people spent their days incessantly searching for food and their nights huddled by a campfire in fear of predators. Because they could never build up food stores, they were always on the verge of starvation—or so went the myth. "It isn't easy to overcome this kind of indoctrination," comments former Columbia University anthropology department chairman George Harris. "Nevertheless . . . much of what we think of as progress is actually a regaining of standards that were widely enjoyed during prehistoric times. . . . The notion that Paleolithic populations worked round the clock in order to feed themselves now also appears ludicrous."[2]

Modern anthropologists have taken to referring to hunter-gatherers as the "original affluent society."[3] Hunter-gatherers ate

more than one hundred species of plants—most rich in vitamins, fiber and other nutrients. They hunted an enormous variety of animals from large game to termites and grubs. Skillfully,
in fact: the bones of one thousand butchered mammoths were
excavated at a single site in Czechoslovakia.[4] This game was all
leaner and higher in protein than anything seen in today's markets and largely free from the diseases of today's farm animals.
The variety of food sources ensured a range of nutrients, and
failure of a single plant or animal could not result in famine.

Our hunter-gatherer ancestors developed their strongest
cravings for nutrients that were essential but rare. Fat was one
such nutrient, meat being leaner and nuts an occasional treat.
Salt, garnered in traces from meat and some vegetables, was
another. Sugar served as a taste cue that other important nutrients were present: it was encountered first in breast milk and
later in fruits and berries. Even sheer calories came to be craved
because high-caloric foods were in scarce supply. Readily available foods such as leafy vegetables were eaten but inspired no
strong cravings.

Despite this "affluent" lifestyle, there were some hard times
during hunter-gatherer evolution. Most notably, forty thousand
years ago, the last Ice Age glaciers began to recede. Mammoths
and other large game retreated toward the poles. Humans followed, dispersing themselves over the world—including their
first venture into the Western Hemisphere. Ultimately, however, the large animals became extinct. Some humans died of
famine as they retreated toward the equator where game herds
of gazelle and deer were still plentiful. Our ancestors were lean
due to their healthy diet and mobile lifestyle, but anyone who
could store energy as modest fat deposits or was inclined to resist
unnecessary exercise had a survival advantage during harsher
times. Therefore, we have developed a hereditary predisposition
for carrying fat on our bodies as well as craving it in our foods.
Until recently it was difficult to get too much.

Modern Hunter-Gatherers

Five hundred years ago, a third of the habitable land still belonged to hunter-gatherers, but this has dwindled to a single-digit percentage occupied by a handful of societies such as the !Kung tribe of Africa.[5] Even in their remaining territory—which is much less lush than the savannah of prehistoric hunter-gatherers—they have a variety of plants and animals from which to choose. The !Kung eat 105 different species of plants and 260 species of animals.

The !Kung walk more than four miles in an average day, carrying hunting equipment and toddlers. Not surprisingly, their cardiovascular fitness, as measured by maximal oxygen uptake, is fully one-third higher than that of the average American. Muscle strength reflects similar differences. Hunter-gatherers' body fat percentages are ideal: 5–15 percent for men, 20–25 percent for women. More remarkably, their body fat does not increase with age. Their average blood pressure is 105/65 (as compared to 120/80 for *young* Americans)—and again, is stable with age. Their blood cholesterol levels average 125 mg/dl. (Americans are advised to keep theirs under 200 mg/dl, but many don't.) Type-2 diabetes is virtually unknown among hunter-gatherers.[6]

!Kung mothers nurse each child for the first two to three years of life. Breast-feeding greatly reduces the chance of pregnancy, so the average interval between !Kung births is 3.7 years[7] and parents can attend generously to each child. The time for leisure and child-rearing is further aided by the fact that hunter-gatherers work only three hours a day for food and shelter.[8] Anthropologists believe this was also true of ancient hunter-gatherers. *Three hours.* Compare that to the hours people work for their food and shelter on a Third World farm *or an American farm.* Compare it to the number of hours expended in a factory *or a law firm* today. The leading experts on hunter-gatherers, anthropologists Richard Lee and Irven DeVore, call this lifestyle "the most successful and persistent adaptation man has ever achieved."[9]

If you still have trouble imagining that early man really had such a leisurely or healthy lifestyle, think of our nearest relatives: the great apes. They eat some meat but more plant food than humans—a slower, more labor-intensive food source. Nevertheless, they spend a modest part of their day foraging and large parts of it playing, napping and interacting with their young. Those bonobos or "pigmy chimps" whose orgiastic sex and idealized society we hear so much about—they're not spending all of their days looking for food (except in areas where humans have completely disrupted their habitat). Our ancestors, with bigger brains and better tools, were more effective foragers yet.

The Agricultural Revolution: "The Worst Mistake in the History of the Human Race"?

Ten thousand years ago, the Paleolithic era ended and the Neolithic "dawn of agriculture" began. Farming is often lauded as a major human advance, but as anthropologists begin to dub hunter-gatherers "affluent," they're coming to view agriculture as correspondingly impoverished. "The Worst Mistake in the History of the Human Race" is the title of an article by historian Jared Diamond, in which he argues, "With agriculture came the gross social and sexual inequality, the disease and despotism, that curse our existence."[10] The ability to accumulate food stores led to huge wealth discrepancies and the origins of warfare, Diamond believes. He traces the origin of problematic gender roles to farming. Farm women weaned babies quickly and spent much more of their lives pregnant—and therefore were much more dependent on men.

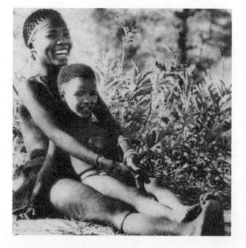

The bush people of the Kalahari live much as hunter-gatherers did in the Paleolithic era. They work three hours a day and enjoy nutritious food and simple shelter with plenty of leisure time for playing with their children. *(Courtesy of I. DeVore, Anthro-Photo)*

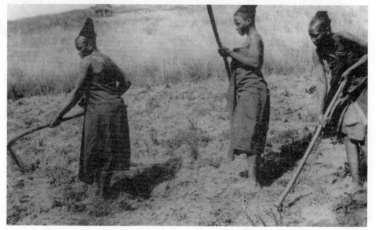

Rural Zulus farm with primitive tools and a limited number of crops, much as the earliest farmers did ten thousand years ago. They toil most of the day to produce food that is deficient in many nutrients. Their work overstrains muscles and joints in wrists and shoulders while failing to provide the aerobic exercise of hunting and gathering. Primitive farmers already suffer from the "diseases of civilization": diabetes, heart disease, arthritis and cancer. *(Courtesy of Pitt Rivers Museum, University of Oxford)*

It's still controversial how many social evils such as war and gender inequality followed directly from farming, and which resulted indirectly from the subsequent crowding of people into denser areas. But there's no doubt about the effect of agriculture on human nutrition, health and fitness. Fossil records show that Paleolithic hunter-gatherers' lifespan averaged twenty-six years. This may sound low today, but with the advent of agriculture it plummeted to nineteen.[11] Most hunter-gatherer deaths were from infectious disease, trauma and childbirth. Those who survived these dangers could expect to live as long as people in industrialized societies today because, as with today's !Kung, there was very little diabetes, heart disease or cancer. Skeletons of early farmers show two categories of increased disease: 1) those unrelated to weight, including a fourfold leap in anemia, three times the rate of osteoporosis, spinal degeneration and infectious disease, more bowel disorders such as appendicitis, diverticulosis, hernias and hemorrhoids; and 2) obesity itself and all the related conditions: diabetes, heart disease and higher rates of cancer[12]

Both types of health problems result directly from changes in diet. Height within any ethnic group is correlated with childhood nutrition. In Greece and Turkey, near the end of the Paleolithic hunter-gatherer era, men averaged 5'9" and women 5'5". By 3000 BC, with agriculture firmly entrenched, heights dropped to 5'3" for men and 5 feet for women. Recently, as a larger variety of foods has been imported, heights have begun to rise, but today's Greeks and Turks haven't yet reached the height of their distant ancestors. Most other areas regained the lost height only very recently. Measurements of early Paleolithic skeletons yield averages of 5'11" for men and 5'6" for women.[13] The current generation of young adults in America is only just reaching this height again. In 1960, the average male in America was still just 5'9".[14] Tooth decay—a health index closely tied to nutrition—shows a similar pattern. In the Paleolithic era, adults died with an average of 2.2 teeth missing; by 6500 BC, with an average of 3.5 missing; and in Roman times, with an average of 6.6 missing (and as we'll get to, this was not due to increased lifespan).

Like the present-day !Kung, Paleolithic hunter-gatherers ate hundreds of plants and animals, supplying generous quantities of complete proteins and vitamins. Farmers switched to a diet determined by which plants were easiest to cultivate, harvest and store without spoiling. Three crops—wheat, rice and corn—provide the bulk of the calories consumed today. These grains are not "natural" foods. They were bred from

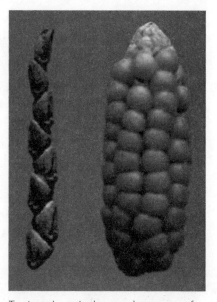

Teosinte, the grain that was the ancestor of all maize and corn. Right: "reconstructed" primitive maize, which resembles the earliest archaeological corn recovered from the Tehuacán Valley in Mexico. It already shows a vastly increased starch content to its kernels and much less fiber, though modern corn is, of course, yet further altered in this direction. *(Photo by John Doebley)*

grasses which produced small seed clusters into plants bearing large, starchy seeds which do not fall off the stalk and germinate. They would die out in one generation if humans did not harvest and replant them. Each of these grains is deficient in at least one essential amino acid and high in simple carbohydrates which promote weight gain. Beyond these three crops, most of the world now eats fewer than twenty other plants.

The earliest farmers had the worst record for illness and lifespan in human history. Scandinavians of this era lived an average of between seventeen and eighteen years.[15] In other parts of Europe, 50–80 percent died as children.[16] When humans began domesticating animals such as cows, pigs and sheep—adding more protein back into farm diets—there was a slight spike upward in human health and lifespan. But this was gradually offset by deaths from new diseases. Illnesses which are thought to have begun as animal diseases—mutating and crossing into humans only when we began to live at close quarters with domestic livestock—include smallpox, tuberculosis, malaria, syphilis, measles and flu.[17]

Got Milk?

For decades, stand-up comics have asked: "What exactly was the first person to realize cows could be milked doing when he discovered this?" The comedian glances to the side slyly. It's actually a discovery that was made around the world, with a variety of animals, presumably simply by seeing animals nurse their young. Sheep, goats, horses, reindeer, water buffalo, yaks and camels have all been domesticated for their milk, though cows now dominate because of their high yield. The only good thing that can be said about feeding babies animal milk is that it was an improvement over the grain mash that was often given to farm babies (and over formulas still in use in the Third World today, which come with instructions to mix with milk but end up water-based through illiteracy or poverty).

Even though it's certainly not sexual, as the stand-up joke implies, there's something just as unnatural in its own way about our milking of cows. No animal's milk has the antibodies most relevant to humans. All have a higher fat ratio than human milk, and all carry some risks of disease. Pasteurizing milk

destroys whatever cow antibodies overlap ours along
with the bacteria it's target-
ing. We now think it bar-
baric if a woman who can't
nurse her child finds a wet
nurse, yet no one pauses to
think it odd that we rou-
tinely use de facto wet
nurses of other species.
Babies fed breast milk average 8.3 IQ points higher by
the age of eight than those
fed milk-based formula,
even after controlling for
the intelligence and edu-
cation of their parents.[18]
The longer babies breast-
feed, the greater the bene-

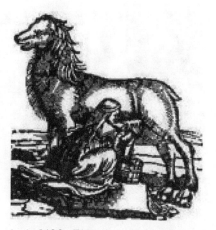

In the 1600s, Tilden depicted the milking
of reindeer by Native Americans in the Far
North to the surprise and amusement of
European settlers. *(Courtesy of Edward
Topsel, in* The History of Four-footed Beasts
and Serpents, *E. Cotes, London, 1607)*

fits. The mechanism by which nutrition affects intelligence is
not completely understood, but researchers believe it has something to do with the requirements of the brain, which completes
90 percent of its development during the first three years.
Human milk matches the exact proportions of amino acids and
fats used for brain circuits and contains antibodies to prevent
infections. Cows' milk contains very different proportions of
amino acids and much more fat. Calves must increase weight at
three times the rate of babies, while their brains are growing
much less. Pasteurized animal milk may allow more frequent illnesses than mothers' milk because of its lack of antibodies—and
these cattle antibodies are only partially matched to human diseases to begin with.

Animal milk isn't a natural food for adults either. It's health-

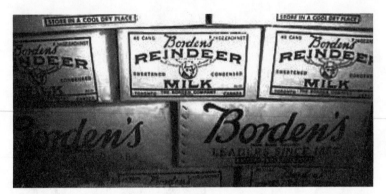

By 1930, Borden's of Canada was canning the same milk. *(Courtesy of Jim Steinborn)*

ier than many modern drinks such as carbonated, sugary sodas. But compared to the water, lean protein and vegetable diet of hunter-gatherer adults, milk is high in saturated fats and calories while low in fiber and many vitamins. And that's before it's turned into higher fat cheese or sugary ice cream.

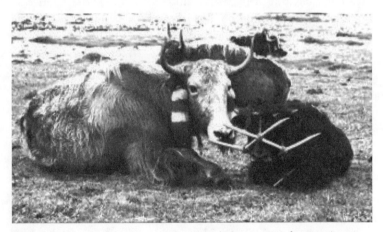

In western Asia, a young yak wears a harness, which prevents it from nursing, reserving the milk for human consumption. *(Courtesy of Magnus Enarsson)*

Survival of the Unfittest?

The dangers to health continue to emerge as the few remaining hunter-gatherer societies switch to farming. A study of the Inuit/Eskimo people finds that diabetes increases *sixty-fold* when they abandon a hunter-gatherer lifestyle and adopt a typical American diet. Cancer and cardiovascular disease also appear when indigenous peoples switch to modern agricultural fare.[19]

The obvious question is: if evolution is defined as "survival of the fittest," how did the less fit farmers take over from the hunter-gatherers? Until fifty years ago, even anthropologists presented farming as an unambiguous advance. It was easy to assume that any change in lifestyle which increased the numbers of a group did so by making "fitter" individuals. It was an evolutionary economist, Elena Boserup, examining why monetary systems which led to massive poverty were nevertheless expanding, who first pointed out the flaw in applying the usual sense of "fitness" to evolution. Darwin's unique definition of fitness is not necessarily what we want for ourselves as individuals, she explained. Evolutionary fitness means passing along the most copies of our genes to offspring who in turn survive to reproductive age.[20] Any additional fitness in terms of individual quality of life, comfort or longevity past that necessary to produce plentiful offspring is irrelevant to evolution.

Once we take into account Boserup's clarification of Darwinian fitness, it's easy to see how agriculture has been good for the human species in terms of sheer numbers. It is indeed when the population explosion began. And yet it's no contradiction to say that the quality of life for most people declined precipitously then.

Babies fed on grain products and other animals' milk were less healthy. In early agricultural societies, children died at higher rates throughout childhood than did children of hunter-gatherers. They did not die at twice the rates, however, and farmers *did* give birth at two to four times the rates of hunter-gatherers. Breast-feeding lowers the chance of getting pregnant even in modern times by changing hormone levels. In Paleolithic times and among the !Kung today, it does so through a second mechanism. On an already low-calorie diet, the extra 1000 calories the nursing infant draws from the mother drop her body fat into a range where pregnancy becomes unlikely.

Farmers' higher-calorie diets also meant that girls reached puberty at thirteen instead of seventeen like the hunter-gatherers—again because body fat promotes fertility while reducing all other health indexes. (Puberty has now dropped to eleven with further increases in calories, estrogen-like pollutants in the environment and the feeding of growth hormones to cattle.) Even with farmers' higher rates of death at every age from infancy onward, their numbers grew faster than hunter-gatherers with their healthier babies, toddlers and adults. Once

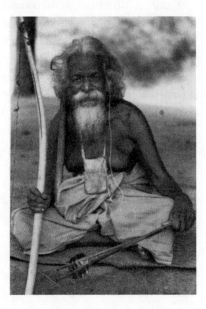

In 1996, Chief Tissahamy of the Veddah ("Forest") People of Sri Lanka successfully petitioned the United Nations to intervene in the confiscation of hunter-gatherer land by the government of Sri Lanka. Chief Tissahamy, who died at age 105 according to his tribe, and at 95 by the estimate of Western anthropologists, illustrates the good health many elderly hunter-gatherers enjoy. *(Courtesy of Wiveca Stegeborn)*

numbers increased, farm acreage needed to expand. Despite hunter-gatherers' better physical fitness, fifty farmers could still drive five hunter-gatherers from their land.

Mind over Mayo

Beginning with Dr. Spock, popular parenting literature has suggested that humans possess "instinctive knowledge" about their nutritional needs. Even some scientists assume this applies to people's eating habits today—ignoring radical changes in our gustatory environment. In one study, which Spock quotes, children chose—on the basis of their own tastes—a variety of healthy foods. But as one critic points out about this research, "The experimental design was poorly constructed, and the children were presented with an array of highly nutritious foods (eggs, milk, cereal, meat, fruits and vegetables). If soft drinks, chocolate, cookies and potato chips had been added to the more nutritious offerings, the results might have been different."[21] Similar studies with adults simply show that they won't eat all fish or all fruit when presented with just these options—not that they won't eat chips, candy and burgers to the exclusion of fish *or* fruit.

Dr. Spock had half the story right: we do possess superb instincts about what to eat—in a hunter-gatherer setting. Unless we put ourselves back in a natural environment—pick vegetables, nuts and berries from fields and forests, and catch fish from streams—we better not simply "listen to our bodies." Evolution hasn't had time to program us with adaptive signals about how to handle fast-food chains and candy shops.

Fortunately, evolution provided us with something else besides these cravings—a giant brain which can sort information and override simple reflex cravings. Predators consistently have larger brains than herbivores; it requires more cunning to

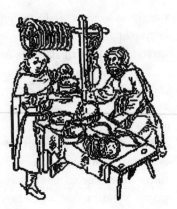

By the fifteenth century, "fast food" stands with greasy, grain-based products could already be found in European cities. *(Fifteenth-century engraving, artist unknown)*

catch prey than to find the next leaf. Omnivores, who must switch between these tasks, tend to have larger brains yet. Hunter-gatherers of the Paleolithic era ate the greatest variety of foods: fruits, berries, vegetables, nuts, roots and prey ranging from insects to animals much larger than themselves—whom they outwitted with their giant brains. Luckily, ten thousand years has not been enough time to devolve our brains to the minimum size needed to locate packaged cupcakes, hamburgers or that fried chicken.

Most animals are guided by absolute cravings. These can be altered by experience; for example, vomiting after eating a particular food can result in a future aversion to it. However, most animals can't learn from others' experience or notice long-term effects on their health. Primates begin to have some simple social learning about foods by observing parents and peers.[22] Humans have the brainpower to elaborate this teaching by verbal and written instructions to each other and can take notice of long-term, not just immediate, effects of a given food on health. Few of us make much use of these abilities today, but the solution to our diet and fitness crisis lies in this ability to learn, not just to operate blindly on obsolete instincts.

What is it we need to learn? *To eat the way we ate ten thousand years ago.* "When, in the interest of preventive medicine, physicians prescribe diet and exercise patterns, they are advocating a way of life generally resembling that of hunter-gatherers," write medical researchers S. Boyd Eaton and Stanley B. Eaton. "It is not by chance that recommendations by groups such as the World Health Organization parallel anthropological findings about the lives of hunters and gatherers."[23]

In the second half of this book, we'll explore how we can eat more like our "affluent" ancestors. We'll consider whether we can reinvent an environment more like the one from which we all sprang so that we can again listen to our bodies. Otherwise we may need to ignore instinctual signals and listen to our intellect. But first, Chapter 3 will detail further deviations from evolution—special maladvances of the last fifty to one hundred years as opposed to those of the previous ten thousand. We'll examine how we've used our big brains to gratify our instinctual cravings in more and more elaborate and self-destructive ways rather than to override them when they lead us astray.

3

Don't Be Too Refined

We usually think of "refinement" as a virtue—not just in manners and culture but even in our foods: silky smooth vichyssoise is favored over chunky potato soup, a French apple tart over the piece of fruit from which it's made. We've become victims of our own sophistication, however. The most dangerous aspect of our modern diet arises from our ability to refine foods. This is the link between overeating and drug, alcohol and tobacco addictions. Coca doesn't give the South American natives dramatic health problems when they brew or chew it. No one has ruined their life eating poppy seeds. When grapes and grains were fermented lightly and occasionally, they presented a healthy pleasure, not a hazard. Salt, fat, sugar and starch aren't harmful in their natural contexts. It's our modern ability to concentrate such things as cocaine, heroin, alcohol—and food components—which turns them into a menace that our body is hardwired to crave.

"Right now, people with substance abuse issues get more respect and better health care treatment," complains a morbidly obese patient in an article on the problems of the heaviest patients.[1] He seems to imply that "substance abusers" deserve the lesser standard of care he's decrying for patients like himself. Of course this isn't true—both groups deserve good health care and basic respect. His perspective is a common one, however: that substance abusers are choosing something bad while obese people are the victims of a disability. *But the obese are "substance abusers."* What could be a more literal definition of the term than ingesting so much of something that your body grows to the size where it can't climb one flight of stairs or fit into an ordinary chair?

Neither hedonistic choice nor genetic fate fully explains any-one's abuse of drugs or nutrients. Substance abuse—including food abuse—is a matter of biological drives, societal habits and personal choices. Almost everyone must exercise some control over cravings. Some people's biochemistry makes that much more difficult—but not impossible. Both drug and food abuse are behaviors that a person can change—albeit through con-certed effort. The model of addictions—especially the concept of the withdrawal period as extremely difficult but brief—can inform fitness strategies. In Chapter 2, we examined how crav-ings arose. Now we'll explore how artificially refined carbohy-drates, fats and minerals interact with these cravings to form addictive patterns.

Too Refined

What we usually mean by "refining" flour, sugar or other foods is removing the hull and fiber, often even the cell wall of plant structures, leaving only simple carbohydrate or clear oil. Before we move on to this standard use of the term, I want to point out how much farming has "refined" our food while it's still on the hoof, leaf or stem. Selective breeding to increase one or more elements which we crave, such as sugar or fat, usually decreases nutrients such as vitamins and fiber. As we've discussed, farmers selected grains that have the largest, starchiest kernels, fruits that have the highest sugar content and farm animals that gain the most weight. Twentieth-century global/industrialized agriculture "refined" raw foods even further. Agronomists sold farmers seeds for bigger, brighter, more regularly shaped, sweeter fruits and vegetables. Foods were also bred to be picked earlier, ripen off the vine and store longer, so that they would still be bigger, brighter and sweeter on the grocery shelves. When demand grew, crops like wheat, iceberg lettuce and bananas were planted on the other side of the world from their native soil.

These priorities select against nutrition—most vitamins and antioxidants taste bitter, not sweet, and don't develop as well unless the food is vine-ripened. They also select against variety when one strain of a vegetable is demonstrably biggest or sweetest or has the longest shelf life. Between 1900 and 2000, 97 percent of existing vegetable and fruit strains went extinct.[2] A recent study of nutrients in food found that, in the second half of that century alone, fruits and vegetables suffered significant decreases in protein, calcium, phosphorus, iron, riboflavin (vitamin B2) and vitamin C. The study concluded that modern agricultural methods designed to improve traits other than nutritive content may be to blame and that there are likely to be similar declines in nutrients which they couldn't study because they weren't reported in 1950, such as fiber, magnesium, zinc, vitamin B6, vitamin E and many other antioxidants.[3] Something very similar happens when we breed animals to be fatter; we automatically decrease their other component, protein.

Probably the only food to ever benefit nutritionally from man's selective breeding is the carrot—and this was completely fortuitous. Carrots were native to Afghanistan and for three thousand years of agricultural history they spread around the world as a whitish root—the color of today's parsnips—with a few variants appearing purple or yellow. About 1600, in Holland, a strain mutated to intense orange just as William the First of Orange was winning freedom from Spain. The Dutch royal chef dedicated the new strain to the monarch and insisted that it be cultivated exclusively.[4] The novel color—created by extra beta-carotene, vitamin A's precursor—caught the eye of the rest of Europe, proving the sole exception to selective breeding sacrificing nutrition.

What we *usually* mean by "refining" has reduced the quality of our diet further while intensifying its addictive potential. Man has been hulling wheat for centuries, but in 1900, 60 percent of it was still whole grain, brown rice was still common and oatmeal was the whole oat that needed to be cooked for half an hour. In the early 1900s, methods for refining food became cheap and virtually all grains began to be stripped of the hulls that contain most of their fiber and much of their protein and vitamins. The fattiest cuts of meat—in which the largest deposits of pure fat had previously been discarded—began to be ground up. The same fat, now mixed back in smaller bits into the meat, made it more appealing. Instead of eating fruit whole, more of it was juiced into bottles for prolonged storage, discarding fiber and oxidizing vitamins. In the last quarter of the century, "juice drinks" containing less than 50 percent juice and more than 50 percent added sugar water became common. High-fructose corn syrup replaced other sugars because corn was cheap to grow, but there were limits to how many ears of corn anyone could consume. It's unclear if corn syrup is actually worse for us than cane sugar, as some argue, but both wreak havoc on insulin/glucose metabolism.[5] Other artificial foods became standard about the same time, such as palm oil and other cheap vegetable oils hydrogenated to resemble animal fat.

Most of these foods look quite unappetizing in their natural states, but with a few cosmetic alterations they're seductive-looking as well as potentially addictive concentrations of sugar and saturated fat. Ground-up animal parts are shaped into pseudo pork chops or even sculpted to imply contours of imaginary underlying bones—check out the patty of the McRib Sandwich. Hydrogenated vegetable oils are dyed yellow to look like the richest butter—margarine would naturally be white.

Many pink, red and purple processed fruit products owe their intense color to an especially bizarre source. The food ingredient listed as "carmine," "carminic acid" or "cochineal extract" is made from the body of the *Dactylopius coccus costa*, a small insect native to Central and South America and the Canary Islands. Several years ago I had the opportunity to visit the studio of Oaxaca weaver Maria Caldones and watched her pick the tiny bugs off prickly pear cacti behind her house and crush them into a bright red dye. This was only slightly disconcerting in Mexico, where the pigment is used to dye yarn for rugs and handspun garments. But I soon learned that this is the same crushed insect which, in Peru and the Canary Islands, is sold to the international food industry to color strawberry yogurt, pink grapefruit drink, and numerous candies and fruit fillings.[6]

Now, I'm not advising you to avoid squashed red bugs, unless you're a committed vegan. Cochineal extract has none of the toxic health effects of most chemical red food colorings and it probably adds traces of protein and minerals to the sugary goo into which it's mixed. You should avoid most of these products for *other* reasons: their sugar content, their excessive calories and their lack of vitamins. It's nevertheless a dramatic commentary on the unnatural places to which our instincts for sweet, red fruit can lead us. To elucidate this phenomenon of why we're drawn to bug-enhanced fruit drinks and sculpted fake ribs, I want to borrow a concept from the field of ethology: that of "supernormal stimuli."

Supernormal Stimuli: Why Birds Are Cuckoo

Ethologist Niko Tinbergen won the 1973 Nobel Prize in biology for his research on instinctive behavior in animals. Tinbergen used various dummies to elicit nurturing, mating and fighting behaviors. He and his students constructed fake eggs which birds would sit on, artificial female butterflies which male butterflies courted and models of male fish which other males attacked. Some of the dummies were ingeniously *unrealistic*, in order to elucidate exactly what characteristics triggered the behaviors. Territorial male stickleback fish will not attack a fish-shaped model if its belly isn't red, but they violently pursue some very unfishlike models when the underside *is* red.

Perhaps the most interesting of Tinbergen's discoveries is that dummies can be devised which surpass the power of any natural stimulus. A male silver-washed fritillary butterfly is more sexually aroused by a butterfly-sized rotating cylinder with horizontal brown stripes than it is by a real, live female of its own kind. Mother birds preferred to try feeding a fake baby bird beak held on a stick by Tinbergen's students if the dummy beak was wider and redder than a real chick's.

Tinbergen coined the phrase "supernormal stimuli" for these dummies that elicit stronger responses than occur naturally. The supernormal stimuli which eventually received the most study were decorated plaster eggs. Tinbergen found that most bird species preferred eggs that were larger than their own and ones which had exaggerated colors or markings. The oyster-catcher, which lays small brown speckled eggs, will ignore them in favor of a giant brown plaster egg the size of the bird itself. Songbirds abandon their pale blue eggs dappled with gray to hop on a black polka-dotted Day-Glo blue dummy so large that they continually slide off and have to climb back on. Ground-nesting birds will retrieve eggs dislodged from the nest, rolling

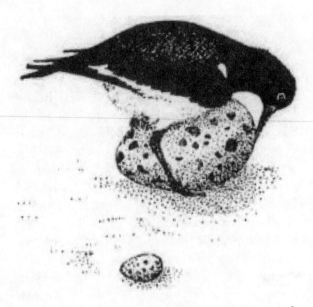

Supernormal stimuli: An oystercatcher abandoning its own egg in favor of an outsize dummy egg. *(After Tinbergen, 1948)*

them back into place. When given a choice between its own egg and a *volleyball*, the greylag goose ignores the egg and tries valiantly to roll the volleyball into the nest.

Tinbergen noted that there's at least one bird which has evolved to be essentially a supernormal stimulus to other species. The cuckoo lays its egg in another bird's nest, where the unsuspecting foster parents incubate and feed it, leaving the mother cuckoo free to fly off to lay more eggs. The baby cuckoo is actually given preferential treatment over the host's offspring. The cuckoo egg is usually larger than the host's, so it is sat on more consistently than the other eggs in the nest. When hatched, the young cuckoo's wider throat acts as a stronger stimulus to the feeding mother than her own chicks'.

The concept of supernormal stimuli is extremely helpful

when thinking about our society's current health woes. Addiction proper is an acquired response which occurs after someone uses heroin, or nicotine, or concentrated sugar enough times to experience withdrawal as the substance drops low in the blood. However, potentially addictive substances appeal to people on first encounter or they'd never be repeatedly ingested enough to be addicting. That's where Tinbergen's concept is relevant. Heroin and high-fructose corn syrup are reinforcing because they're intensified versions of natural endorphins and natural glucose levels respectively—very much like what Tinbergen meant by supernormal stimuli. Even more analogous to Tinbergen's dummies, the exaggeration of visual elements in addictive foods often plays a role in hooking us. Keep in mind the image of that bird sliding off the giant polka-dot egg while we examine the rise of the bacon double cheeseburger. I will return to it repeatedly in later chapters as we examine the lure of television and spectator sports.

Food as Drug

What happens when we eat these supernormally stimulating, highly refined foods? With simple carbohydrates, glucose levels soar in the bloodstream. In the short term, our bodies release insulin to store the glucose as fat. In the long term, we respond to this high level of insulin with decreasing sensitivity to it— developing diabetes in which blood sugar levels remain elevated, causing damage to our kidneys, eyes and immune system. Possibly the worst aspect of these foods is that we can happily eat a lot before our bodies register that we're full; very soon, as glucose levels plummet, they trigger hunger again.

There is growing evidence that sugary foods can trigger changes in the same brain chemicals affected by addictive drugs. Researchers at Princeton have shown that natural opioids are released when rats eat a large amount of sugar and that they're thrown into a state of anxiety when the sugar is removed. Symptoms included chattering teeth and the shakes—very similar to those seen in people withdrawing from nicotine or morphine. When the rats were given naloxone, a drug that blocks opioid receptors, dopamine levels dropped and acetylcholine increased. This is the neurochemical pattern shown by heroin addicts as they go into opioid withdrawal.[7] "The implication is that some animals—and by extension some people—can become overly dependent on sweet food," writes study author John Hoebel. "The brain is getting addicted to its own opioids as it would morphine or heroin. Drugs give a bigger effect, but it's essentially the same process."[8]

Biologists are also finding that overeating refined fatty meals triggers similar physiological changes. Leptin is a hormone which signals the body to stop eating after a certain point when consuming natural foods. When researchers at Albert Einstein Medical College fed rats unnaturally fatty meals, however, after just a few such meals the animals lost almost all of their ability to respond to leptin. They just kept eating.[9] Fortunately the effect reversed when they were taken off the high fat for a while.[10] A study at Rockefeller University offers more evidence that a high-fat diet reconfigures the body's hormonal system to want yet more fat. Galanin, a brain peptide that increases eating and slows energy expenditure, rises in rats on a high-fat diet. In fact, it only takes one high-fat meal to stimulate galanin release and the craving of more fat. When the effects of galanin are blocked chemically, the animals eat much less fat. "The peptide is itself responsive to the consumption of fat, which then creates the basis for a vicious cycle," writes lead researcher Sarah Leibowitz.[11]

One especially bad category of fats, trans fats, is produced by heating liquid vegetable oils in the presence of metal catalysts and hydrogen. This gives them a different shape from either the original oil or the natural saturated fats found in meat. They don't fit properly with cell membranes or with enzymes designed to digest fats. Trans fats cause a significant drop in HDL (good) cholesterol and a significant increase in LDL (bad) cholesterol,[12] they make veins and arteries more rigid, they cause major clogging of arteries[13] and they generally contribute to the risk of death from heart disease.[14] Because trans fats contain abundant calories without providing the beneficial fats found in natural vegetable oil, they lead to overeating with undernutrition. Trans fats now make up much of the fat in candy, commercial cookies and cakes, and the oils in which fast-food chains fry food.

The number of calories people consume has risen drastically. A recent study in the *American Journal of Clinical Nutrition* based on data from the US Department of Agriculture and Centers for Disease Control found that Americans had increased their average daily intake by 500 calories since 1980, and that "Specifically, 428 calories (nearly 80 percent of the increase in total energy) came from carbohydrates." The bulk—the grams—of carbohydrate foods hasn't changed much but the carbohydrate calories have; instead of whole grains and vegetables, people are getting more and more of those carbs from processed grains and sugars. Even the touted reduction in our fat consumption isn't real—the *percentage* of calories derived from fat has declined only because the amount of fat Americans eat has risen less than the amount of carbohydrates. The authors of the study pointed out that this increase in total calories and especially carbs closely parallels the rise in the number of cases of type-2 diabetes.[15]

Another study in the *Journal of Food Chemistry and Analysis* examined in more detail exactly where our calories are coming from, and found that 25 percent were from completely nonnutritive sources. Candy, other desserts, soft drinks and alcoholic beverages account for a quarter of all calories consumed by

Americans. Even more came from foods such as burgers, fries and pizza that have some nutrients, but in meager proportion to their calorie counts. "In contrast, such healthy foods as vegetables and fruit make up only 10 percent of the caloric intake in the US diet. A large proportion of Americans are undernourished in terms of vitamins and minerals." The authors concluded, "You can actually be obese and still be undernourished with regard to important nutrients."[16]

The standard portion size for almost everything is larger than it was a generation ago. People are conscious of this in restaurants, but often unaware that they're serving more at home, too. Do you know that even the size of plates is larger? Antique collectors find that many old china cabinets won't close with modern plates on their shelves, and modern salad plates have begun to equal the dimensions of antique dinner plates. You're probably eating off a plate a couple of inches larger than what your parents served your food on.

There's a Woody Allen joke about a woman criticizing a restaurant. "Their food is terrible," she complains, "and their servings are so small, too!" In a research experiment eerily reminiscent of the joke, the University of Illinois Food and Brand Lab offered free popcorn to moviegoers at a $1 movie theater. Half the audience was given fresh popcorn, either in small containers or jumbo buckets; the other half received fourteen-day-old stale popcorn in small or jumbo containers. Even though 82 percent of the people with the old popcorn reported it tasted terrible, those with the jumbo buckets ate 33 percent more of it than those with the smaller containers. People with the fresh popcorn also ate more from the larger size.[17] The fat, salt, carbs and appealing appearance of the popcorn make it a supernormal stimulus *even without a pleasing taste*—and the large container accentuates this.

The Food and Brand Lab has demonstrated the effect of larger portions on consumption in a variety of situations. They found that cooks used more of both liquid Crisco and dry spaghetti when pouring from containers that were jumbo-sized than when pouring from smaller containers.[18] In another experiment, students were invited to the lab for a "taste test" of soup. Some got trick "bottomless" bowls of soup rigged with hidden tubes that kept them full as the students ate, while others had regular bowls. Those with bottomless bowls ate 40 percent more than subjects with regular bowls.[19]

"Don't snack now or you'll spoil your appetite for supper," our mothers used to warn us. But is this true? There's some evidence that when people eat high-fiber, slow-to-digest food, it decreases the calories they will eat at the next meal. But these are hardly the usual snacks. Unfortunately, salty tidbits and sweets don't spoil our appetite. In yet another study of portion size, people given sugary drinks drank more from a large serving than a small—and then ate the same amount of supper later whether they'd drunk the small portion, the large, or a control condition of no-calorie artificially sweetened drinks.[20] Nor do people adjust for excess calories over longer periods of time. Subjects told researchers that they usually gained weight during the December holidays and took it off in the later winter and spring. Only the first half of this proved true. Experimenters followed these subjects for a year, weighing them at weekly intervals. They indeed added several pounds in December—but eleven months later most still carried the extra weight.[21]

You Are What You Drink

I've been discussing mostly what people eat, but, as the sugary drink study suggests, many of our calories come in liquid form. In 2006, soda, juice, milk, beer and other beverages accounted for 21 percent of the calories consumed by Americans, up from 16 percent in the 1970s.[22] Soft drinks make up the largest number of these calories for adults, with most of them coming straight from diabetes-inducing sugar. There is some controversy about whether soft drinks sweetened with corn sweeteners (half fructose) are worse than those sweetened with cane sugar (mostly sucrose), but there's no disagreement among researchers that both are very, very bad for health.

Diet drinks contain no sugar and virtually no calories and have been assumed to be healthier. This was questioned at the 2006 meeting of the American Diabetes Association, where researchers presented a disturbing finding on diet soft drinks and their correlation with weight. People who drink diet soft drinks don't lose pounds on average—they gain. There was a 41 percent increase in the risk of being overweight for every can or bottle of diet soft drink a person consumed per day. This was much higher than the risk from drinking regular, i.e., sugar-laden, soft drinks.[23]

Most experts don't think this means that artificial sweeteners cause obesity. They think it is likelier that consumption of diet soft drinks is a marker for obesity—something that correlates with it for other reasons. This view assumes that people see they are beginning to gain weight and switch to diet soda but don't make other necessary changes. People mistake diet drinks for diets, says sports nutritionist Leslie Bonci. "You can't go into a fast-food restaurant and say, 'Oh, it's okay because I had diet soda.' If you don't do anything else but switch to a diet soft drink, you are not going to lose weight."[24]

There is another, more sinister explanation. Researcher Sharon Fowler suggests "the Mad Hatter theory," named for a scene in *Alice in Wonderland*:

> "Take some more tea," the March Hare said to Alice, very earnestly.
> "I've had nothing yet," Alice replied in an offended tone, "so I can't take more."

"You mean you can't take *less*," said the Hatter: "It's very easy to take more than nothing."[25]

Alice is offered tea but given none, so she eventually helps herself to tea *and* bread and butter. That may be what happens when we taste artificial sweeteners. "If you offer your body something that tastes like a lot of calories, but it isn't there, your body is alerted to the possibility that there is something there and it will

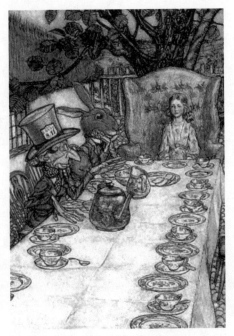

(© British Library Board. Bridgeman Art Library)

search for the calories promised but not delivered," Fowler says.[26]

One study of saccharine reported that, after drinking it, rats ate three times as much as when they drank sugar water.[27] However, a small study published in the March 2006 issue of *Pediatrics* found the opposite—that overweight teenage boys lost weight when their soft drinks were replaced with calorie-free drinks.[28] If you're having trouble losing weight, it might be worth trying whatever drink strategy you haven't yet explored—adopt or drop or switch artificial sweeteners. The jury is still out on this. Answers may prove to be different for the varied chemicals currently used as sweeteners. You can certainly never go wrong with the drink of the hunter-gatherers: water.

The Immigrant Advantage

My Russian immigrant friend Olga Michnikov was the first person to point out to me the kind of people who shop in the farmers' markets of Boston—and it turns out to be similar around the country. Other than buyers for restaurants, the most typical customers are recent immigrants. When Olga moved here three decades ago she was part of a wave of Jews leaving Russia, and they were the ones who frequented the markets. Now it's Southeast Asians. Recent immigrants are often on limited budgets and looking for bargains—but they're also looking for fresh produce rather than the prepared foods that fill so many US grocery shelves.

Immigrants do well to avoid American eating habits. Immigrants are more likely to be poor and less likely to visit a doctor regularly—two factors usually correlated with shorter lifespan. However, research at the National Institutes of Health (NIH) finds that immigrants live an average of three years longer than people born here.[29] Immigrant life expectancy surpasses seventy-eight, while US-born life expectancy hovers around seventy-five. The effect is significant for all categories of immigrants, but it's strongest among minorities who have the lowest American life expectancies and greater for men than women. The largest differences are for immigrant black men who live *nine years longer* than black men born in the United States—seventy-three versus sixty-four years. The difference is not as simple as the country of origin being all-round healthier. Researchers estimated that the same African-born man remaining in his homeland would probably have died before his fiftieth birthday. Long-term habits are better in most other countries—eating unprocessed food, getting more exercise, drinking and smoking less. When someone continues these practices after moving to the US, with its lower rates of infectious disease, war and famine—and better emergency healthcare—it's a winning combination.

The NIH researchers concluded that weight was a major link between lifestyle factors and varying lifespans. Twenty-two percent of adult immigrants were obese, compared to 28 percent of US-born adults. The longer people had been here, the higher the rate of obesity. "Assimilation often means assimilation into eating too much Cheez Whiz," observed Mark Krikorian, director of the Center for Immigration Studies.[30]

McHunters and McGatherers

In a *New York Times* satire, Nicholas Kristof describes spotting a 6'5" figure in a burka while checking email at a Kandahar Starbucks. The imaginary interview with Osama bin Laden reads in part:

> Q: So what's your strategic aim? To kill lots of Americans?
> A: No. If we wanted to do that, we'd have our agents open up McDonald's franchises . . .[31]

Fast food is so universally understood to be unhealthy that no one needs the joke explained. McDonald's is the most popular target for such jabs if only because it's the largest, "supersize" target. In April 2004, Morgan Spurlock released his documentary film *Super Size Me*, in which he gained 25 pounds, 60 points of cholesterol and a fatty liver in just one month of eating exclusively McDonald's food. Three months later, denying it had anything to do with Spurlock's film, McDonald's announced that they were phasing out their "Supersize that?" promotional campaign. In the early 1990s, they ran an even more intensive advertising campaign, the "Big Mac attack"—a series of vignettes about people overcome by an irresistible urge to consume their product. In 1992, journalists used the phrase in covering a woman's collapse from anaphylactic shock after a rare allergic reaction to a Big Mac. The term cropped up in numerous cartoons about heart attacks. McDonald's discontinued the "Big Mac attack" ads, again denying any relation to the new connotations.

But McDonald's survived—even thrived—in the face of negative publicity. The years 1990–94 saw the "McLibel" trial—the longest-running lawsuit in the history of the British legal system. McDonald's brought charges against two Greenpeace activists for distributing a pamphlet called "What's Wrong with McDonald's?" After spending $10 million in legal fees against the two defendants, who served as their own counsel, McDonald's won . . . technically. The defendants were found liable for $78,000 in damages because the court judged them not to have proved all of the claims in the pamphlet. The court did deem them to have proved that McDonald's "exploited children" with their ads and endangered the health of its regular customers. The defendants appealed, and in the new hearing the judge ruled that they had also proven that McDonald's food can cause heart disease. Some allegations were still judged unproven and libelous—mainly statements about mistreatment of their workers rather than about health hazards of their product.[32] McDonald's chose to withdraw the suit at this point. Pundits pronounced this a public relations disaster, but McDonald's continued to increase profits throughout the period—including from its British franchises. The non-health-related problems with McDonald's and other food chains are outside the scope of this book, but substandard working conditions at some McDonald's and the fast-food industry settlement of sexual harassment suits with distinctive twists such as "explicit use of animal parts" are colorfully described in Eric Schlosser's *Fast Food Nation*.[33]

McDonald's customers are not the only people who should

worry about the health effects of burgers and fries. In the spring of 2004, as *Super Size Me* was showing in America's theaters, McDonald's CEO was James Cantalupo, age sixty, a thirty-year veteran of the company. Cantalupo was at the helm through the McLibel trial and was famous for consuming the product in public. On April 19, he dropped dead of a heart attack at a McDonald's franchisee convention in Orlando, Florida. Literally within hours, the company appointed a successor: forty-three-year-old Australian Charlie Bell, who'd begun his McDonald's career flipping burgers and mopping floors at age fifteen and worked his way up to the top spot. Seven months after becoming CEO, Bell was diagnosed with colon cancer—another disease whose incidence rises with a diet high in fat and red meat and low in fiber. Bell died four months later. McDonald's news releases discussed the financial and organizational impact of two successive losses, but studiously avoided any mention of public relations or health implications.

So is McDonald's any worse than the rest of the fast-food chains? No—or only to the extent that it's doing more business so it's doing more harm. McDonald's is the largest owner of retail property in world.[34] Seven percent of American adults eat at McDonald's in a given day—and 96 percent of us eat there at least once a year. Several years ago, McDonald's replaced Coke as the world's most famous brand.[35] After decades of scoring high 90-something percents on name recognition for its company mascot, Ronald McDonald (consistently higher than any other figure, including Jesus), the latest poll found the clown had "virtually 100 percent recognition" in the US, with 98 percent in Japan and 93 percent in the UK (probably *aided* by the McLibel trial).[36] The magazine *Advertising Age* named Ronald McDonald the number two advertising icon of the twentieth century, followed closely by the Green Giant, Betty Crocker, the Pillsbury Doughboy, Aunt Jemima, Tony the Tiger and Elsie the Cow—giving food companies seven of the top ten slots. But they didn't capture number one; that honor went to the Marlboro Man.

In everything except recognition, McDonald's competitors are similar or worse. Despite the jokes about Big Mac Attacks, a Big Mac with cheese at 560 calories and 30 grams of fat (half the recommended daily allotment) doesn't set any records (even McDonald's features a Double Quarter Pounder with Cheese at 730 calories and 40 grams of fat). The largest burger at any major chain for many years was Burger King's Double Whopper with Cheese at 1,070 calories and 70 grams of fat. It was recently bested by Hardee's Monster Thickburger at 1,420 calories and 107 grams of fat. The Center for Science in the Public Interest, a Washington-based nonprofit nutritional education group, termed these oversized burgers "food porn." (I'd note that pornography itself is a supernormal stimulus.) CSPI called Hardee's Monster Thickburger "the fast-food equivalent of a snuff film."[37]

A *St. Petersburg Times* column noted that there were healthier lunches than Monster Thickburger—one could "have a stick of butter instead. That has only 800 calories and 88 grams of fat. We could always wrap it in bacon." In a skit on *The Late Show*, David Letterman questioned an actor playing the CEO of Hardee's about the health risks of a burger the size of the Monster; the faux CEO clutched his chest and keeled over—eerily reminiscent of Cantalupo's demise. How does the real Hardee's CEO answer that question? "Not every product has to be aimed at the health-conscious," Andy Puzder told the Associated Press, noting that since the introduction of the Thickburger family in April 2003, sales for the 2,067-restaurant chain have risen steadily and that sales for the Monster specifically "have exceeded all expectations."[38]

It's not only in food chains, of course, that we find junk food or oversized concoctions. The plastic-wrapped subs and burritos at many convenience stores exceed the Monster's calories and fat; standard grocery stores are filled with huge bags of candy and chips, cookie bits masquerading as cereal and 4,000-calorie frozen pizzas. It bears repeating that fast food and the ubiquitous advertisements for it don't *cause* our dangerous dietary inclinations, they just aggravate them. Our instincts are already out of sync with our food production technology. We need to use our intellect to overcome the biologically driven trap of supernormally stimulating refined food—not simply to figure out that eating in fast-food chains isn't smart. An important point that I'll get back to in Chapter 9 is that the fast-food chains are not out to kill us, as in the bin Laden satire quoted above; they're out to make as much money as possible. Chains would cooperate and make money from healthy veggies if demand changed enough. But demand isn't changing. Chain attempts at lighter fare such as the McLean burger and Taco Bell's Border Lights were discontinued due to lack of sales. "It's well known in the food service industry that the best way to kill the success of a new product is to put a heart symbol [indicating it's low-fat] next to it on the menu," says food marketing researcher John Stanton. "And I can certainly tell you that their customers aren't saying they want smaller portions or are ordering Big Macs and fries and asking about trans fats. They don't want these healthier options."[39]

Junk Food Junior

"The Pester Factor," "The Fine Art of Whining" and "Why Nagging Is a Kid's Best Friend" are all titles of articles written not to help parents to curb whining but to teach advertisers how best to provoke it. Advertising to children has become big business— nowhere more so than in the fast-food industry. McDonald's 1997 Teenie Beanie Baby give away was named "one of the most successful promotions in the history of American advertising" by *Brandweek*. McDonald's was already selling ten million Happy Meals a week. In the ten days of that promotion, they sold one hundred million. Happy Meals target children aged three to nine, so this translates into three to four meals for every child in that age range.[40]

Unhappily, the number of overweight children in America has tripled in the last three decades. This is directly related to an increase in their junk-food consumption. One-third of American children eat at fast-food restaurants every day. These children average a daily intake of 187 calories more than other children, which results in an extra six pounds a year assuming equal exercise. And while the children's menus at fast-food restaurants are as unhealthy as the adults', at the sit-down chains the kids' offerings are *worse* than the adults'. The Center for Science in the Public Interest surveyed menus at the largest twenty chain restaurants in the United States, including Applebee's, Chili's, Cracker Barrel, Denny's, Olive Garden and Outback Steakhouse. They found that adult offerings usually included grilled chicken entrées and sides of vegetables and salads, but the children's menus featured mainly fried entrées which were automatically accompanied by French fries and a dessert.[41]

And our schools? "7-Elevens with books," is how Yale diet expert Kelly Brownell describes them.[42] Fast-food franchises such as Pizza Hut are manufacturing many of their offerings and even running their lunch rooms. The old-fashioned hot-food cafeteria lines now serve pizza and spaghetti and burgers no more nutritious than those of the chains anyway. "We try to be more like the fast-food places where the kids are hanging out," one administrator explained. "We want kids to think of school lunch as a cool thing, the cafeteria as a cool place, that we're with it, that we're not institutional."[43] Can you imagine canceling algebra and world history and substituting courses on the private lives of rock stars because kids judge this more cool?

The film *Super Size Me* dramatically illustrates how children are actually eating at school. Spurlock filmed kids buying com-binations of chips, fries, cake and soft drinks in a school cafete-ria line. On camera, the cafeteria director assured him they were fetching side orders for a whole table of friends who'd brought standard entrées from home. But when Spurlock followed the kids to the table, guess what? They were indeed making meals of the snacks—any food they'd brought from home was usually additional sodas or desserts.

When children bring lunch from home, it's more and more likely to be processed, prepared foods. Perhaps the most popular item for the school lunchbox is Kraft Foods' Lunchables. In 1988, when these debuted, all were under 300 calories. By 2003, Kraft was making Mega Pack Lunchables like "Deep Dish Pizza—Extra Cheesy" with 640–780 calories.

Before and after lunch, vending machines are available—full of chips, candy and sugary sodas. In a recent survey, 67 percent of kids report that they buy junk food or soda from vending machines at school. Seventy-five percent of overweight kids do so. And it's very difficult to get bans on these vending machines.[44] Soft-drink and snack-food companies sponsor increasing numbers of school sporting events and have consid-erable influence with school boards and administrators.

In 2006, after years of thwarted proposals grew closer to pas-sage, the major beverage venders voluntarily agreed to remove sodas from machines in elementary schools and junior highs—there they will sell only bottled water, juices and milk. In high schools, they will still sell carbonated diet drinks and sugar-laden "sports drinks"—but no longer drinks that are both car-bonated and sugar-laden.[45] As we discussed with the Mad Hatter theory, it's not clear whether diet drinks are diet-friendly either. In Chapter 9 we'll discuss further initiatives needed for food machines and hot meal programs in schools.

In *Kids as Customers: A Handbook of Marketing to Children*, advertising guru James McNeal outlines the reasons restaurant and food brands focus so intently on children: first, they're good immediate customers; second, they influence their parents' eating habits; and third, there's "brand loyalty"—the concept that they'll grow into adults who'll prefer their childhood food brands. Within the industry, fast-food chains refer to their regular customers as "heavy users" in their internal communications, though they assiduously avoid leaking the term into the public sphere because they recognize it has both obesity and addiction connotations.[46]

Overseas

The reason Japanese people are so short and have yellow skins is because they have eaten nothing but fish and rice for two thousand years. If we eat McDonald's hamburgers and potatoes for a thousand years, we will become taller, our skin will become white, and our hair will be blond.

—Den Fujita,
CEO of Japanese McDonald's for three decades[47]

"He can't really have said that," was my first thought when I saw this quote in a recent muckraking book about McDonald's, "or he must have been joking." In tracking it down, however, I found Fujita actually made remarks to this effect numerous times in talks and press conferences in the year he opened Japan's first McDonald's restaurant three decades ago. He wasn't joking, though it's not clear if he believed it. One of *Forbes*'s "Richest People in the World" consistently until his death in 2004, Fujita was known to have held some very eccentric beliefs but also to have intentionally courted publicity with great flamboyance.[48] And *one* of his three claims is true. If a population that has been eating modest servings of fish and rice suddenly switches to eating large orders of hamburgers and fries, the children of that generation will become taller than their parents and grandparents. Sheer calories in childhood have some effect on height, and artificial bovine growth hormone—now found routinely in hamburger—augments this effect. Asians are getting *a bit* taller as they adopt Western eating habits—and as they get *much* fatter for the same reason.[49]

While Fujita ramped his net worth to over $1 billion selling Big Macs and fries to his compatriots, other foreign franchisers tried adapting McDonald's menus to their countries' traditional foods. The Australian outlets sold English-style fish and chips—with little success. "McDonald's had better luck changing the local eating habits than adapting its menu to fit them," observed financial analyst John Love.[50] Registering this lesson, the first golden arches in England opened with American-style fries. They touted these as "crispy," with the clear implication that British "Chips" were soggy.

McDonald's met with rapid success in its new locales. During my 1973 undergraduate semester studying in Paris, I observed French haute couture shoppers lining up by the hundreds outside the newly opened golden arches on the Champs-Elysées. Decades later, I traveled to Kuwait in the wake of the Iraqi occupation to teach Kuwaiti psychologists about trauma therapy and watched their first McDonald's open to similar crowds.

McDonald's and other Western chains do run into the occasional cross-cultural problem, but when they do it's not a matter of the taste of their supernormal stimuli, but of religious or political insensitivity. "Welcome to Dachau," read leaflets distributed to cars in the parking lot of the Dachau Memorial Museum, "and welcome to McDonald's." After the curator of the museum complained, the leaflets were discontinued. Jewish groups continue to protest the presence of the franchise, which is built on ground once tilled by concentration camp inmates.[51] An article in the *New York Times* titled "Where's the Beef? It's in Your Fries"[52] precipitated a class-action lawsuit in this country and the flinging of cow dung at a Bombay McDonald's.[53] The fries were originally crisped in lard; now they are done in vegetable oil with added "beef extract." Neither is what a customer on a vegetarian diet assumes.

When US troops entered Iraq, McDonald's experienced calls for boycotts and suffered numerous acts of vandalism around the Middle East. Most American-based chains had problems—except Pizza Hut, whose relieved CEO speculated, "I guess they think we're Italian." McDonald's responded to the anti-American sentiment by introducing ethnically themed variations of its products, such as the McArabia sandwich—basically a Big Mac on Middle Eastern flatbread. McDonald's denied permission to reproduce the McArabia advertisements in this book, along with a series declaring: "My Ramadan has a special taste." The latter depicts Moslems waiting longingly for sunset, when they will be able to indulge in a McDonald's strawberry custard pie free with each Supersize meal through Ramadan. Similarly, McDonald's will not allow readers to see its European billboard featuring no text other than its trademark arches and picturing a baby sucking on a hamburger bun oriented to look like a female breast. Such cynical humor is appreciated in Europe but might be off-putting to both American and Middle Eastern customers. These ads are posted on the Web, where they are often mistaken by Americans for Photoshopped parodies.

These culture-specific campaigns have been largely successful; McDonald's and other chains have expanded to include Iraq itself. An Aljazeera cartoon ran shortly after the invasion depicting a television showing news of American military action. On an oriental carpet in front of it sits an Arab man shaking one fist at the screen while clutching a McDonald's cheeseburger in the other.

Some think the popularity of McDonald's, Burger King and Pizza Hut around the world lies in a glamorous American cachet—and there's some truth to that. But there's also a deep animosity toward America in much of the world, as demonstrated by the attacks on franchises. I think the phenomenal success lies largely with what McDonald's and other chains are selling. One might think of the old joke definition of heaven and hell by nationality: In heaven the administration is Swiss, the police force is British, the auto mechanics are German, the lovers are Italian and the chefs are French; in hell, the administrators are Italian, the police are German, the auto mechanics French, the lovers Swiss and the chefs British. Americans aren't mentioned at all in this joke, but it's American chains that have tossed aside the soggy British chips and replaced them with "French fries"—crispy like *pommes frites* but with the added stimulus of meat seasoning. The major fast-food products are remarkably similar—chains have taken products from disparate countries and shaped them toward identical ratios of refined carbohydrate, saturated fat and salt—and then served them in huge portions. These are followed by desserts with similar refined carbs and fats but with sugar substituted for salt and meat flavoring—essentially the same ratios, albeit with much cheaper ingredients, that French pastry has long contained. Fast foods the world over show few variations from the formula. McArabia bread only *looks* different from hamburger buns. Some Asian fast food still features totally refined rice instead of wheat, but it's mixed into virtually identical portions of fat and either sugar or salt.

Fast-food restaurants have perfected the supernormal stimulus—and it's spreading around the world like a virus. In more and more locales, the obese are up against a situation similar to that of the heroin addict living in a neighborhood with a pusher on every corner. In Chapter 8 I'll describe what an individual can do within this environment, and in Chapter 9 I'll explore what a society can do as a whole to change this back to a healthy environment. But first, in Chapters 4 through 7, we'll explore just what weight and fitness goals we should be seeking—beginning with exercise in Chapter 4.

4

Get a Move On

The sea squirt is a tube-shaped organism that lives in colonies rooted to the ocean floor or the hulls of ships. It has long been an overgrowth nuisance in Britain and is now spreading at alarming rates off the coast of Maine and Canada. It presents no problem in France or Japan, where it's enthusiastically harvested and sautéed or consumed raw with lemon juice.

The sea squirt gets its name from its feeding process—sucking in seawater, extracting plankton, bacteria and algae, and expelling the filtered water forcefully. Its scientific name, *Ciona intestinalis*, evokes a similar image—a large, freestanding intestine. The adult sea squirt is immobile and has no sensory organs or central nervous system. It's such a primitive animal that it could easily be mistaken for a plant. In fact, its feeding tube is composed of cellulose, a fiber typically produced by plants and bacteria, which no other multicelled animal manufactures.

Remarkably, the sea squirt begins life as a more complex organism. Larvae bud off from the parent, grow muscular tails and swim like tadpoles. At this stage of life, the sea squirt has an eye, a balance organ—and, most importantly, a rudimentary brain and nervous system. Squirts navigate the ocean looking for a new home. Upon finding one, they attach themselves. They never move again.

Within thirty minutes, their muscles begin to be re-absorbed. The rudimentary brain, nerve cord and sensory organs are also absorbed—recycled to build the rapidly expanding digestive tract. One lone neuronal node remains, to control the rhythmic sucking and expelling of nutrient-rich water. Squirts need their nervous systems only for movement. This is why the adult squirt resembles a plant so closely. Brains and nervous systems are for mobility; plants don't have brains, animals do. With a few other exceptions, animals move, plants don't.

Sea squirts are not even relatives of the simplest animals. They're more closely related to fish, birds and people than to worms, starfish or other invertebrates. Like humans, squirts belong to a group of animals called chordates, meaning they have spinal cords. Their sperm and eggs are so like ours that they're now being harvested to search for "activating factor"— a protein in sperm which initiates cell division once an egg is

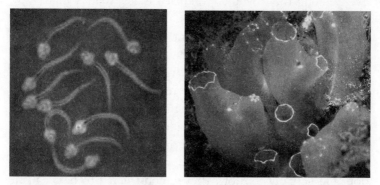

The sea squirt (*Ciona intestinalis*) begins life as a tadpolelike organism with a rudimentary brain, central nervous system, sensory organs and a muscular tail. When it finds its permanent home, it attaches itself to a rock and digests both muscle and brain—turning into one large intestine. *(Photos courtesy of DOE Joint Genome Institute)*

fertilized. This area of infertility research was previously done only with human tissue.[1]

Most of evolution has progressed from simpler to more complex organisms, so it's remarkable to see one that developed a nervous system and movement and then retreated from these adaptations. Genes switching on and off at different stages of life is a well-known phenomenon; however, this usually results in subtler modifications than those of squirts—more typically a growth hormone manufactured at one age and not another.

All of this suggests the whimsical possibility that humans may be encoded with a DNA switch which, if activated, would cause us to attach ourselves to the nearest surface, digest our brains and do nothing but eat for the rest of our lives. Or perhaps this has already happened?

The Principle of Least Effort

Ninety percent of Americans travel to work in personal vehicles. Even among those whose workplace is less than a mile away, only 25 percent bike or walk—half the number who did just twenty years ago.[2] Fifteen percent of people get the minimum amount of *vigorous* activity recommended by US Department of Health guidelines: three times a week for at least twenty minutes. Twenty-two percent get the recommended amount of *light to moderate* exercise: walking five times a week for at least thirty minutes. Twenty-five percent of adults report they do no physical activity at all in their leisure time.[3] Many trainers, medical researchers and evolutionary biologists say these recommendations are actually too low; they're constructed to be "realistic expectations" and not to scare people off.[4] Yet even these mild recommendations are too much for most of us.

Three-quarters of Americans think they should get more exercise. The most common reason cited for not doing so is too little time. Modern "time-saving" devices don't work; "labor-saving" ones unfortunately do. People also report that they don't exercise due to health complaints such as shortness of breath or knee pain. Ironically, most of these problems are improved by exercise rather than by avoiding it. Others worry that going out to exercise makes them or their children more vulnerable to crime. We'll say more about all of these issues later in the chapter, in terms of which priorities our Paleolithic programming overemphasizes in the modern environment.

The basic problem is that biologically we need exercise, but we don't have strong instincts to engage in it. Physical activity used to occur automatically while seeking food, shelter and friends, and in taking care of children. Lower animals do seem

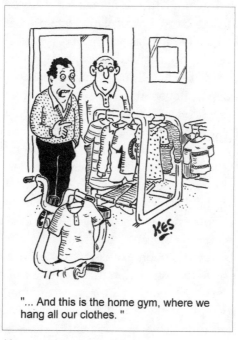

"... And this is the home gym, where we hang all our clothes."

(Courtesy of www.CartoonStock.com)

to have instincts to exercise. If you place a wheel in the cage of a mouse or rat, it never goes unused. Place a stair-climber or treadmill in a human's apartment and the results are less predictable. There is more sitting and less action in a zoo's ape house than in an aquarium, aviary or insect exhibit. Humans have more choice in their behavior; this gives us greater flexibility but more responsibility for figuring out and adopting healthy lifestyles.

A principle articulated in 1949 provides another perspective on this, in statistical rather than evolutionary terms. George Zipf's *Human Behavior and the Principle of Least Effort* describes how—across a wide variety of endeavors—people do what's easiest, not what's best. Zipf observed that most people, most of the time, are turned back by modest hurdles that they know could be overcome with effort. "To be habitual, an action must be relatively effortless or carry a particularly large psychic reward," he observed. Originally Zipf was writing about word usage. But his ideas have recently been applied to statistical analyses of Internet behavior, and Zipf believed his principle applied to all human activity. The most important aspect of his observation was that what constitutes a "large reward" can be either instinctual or intellectually deduced and is definitely amenable to learning.[5]

Right now most people are caught in a vicious cycle of not exercising, which makes them less energetic and therefore even less inclined to exercise. However, the same mechanisms that contribute to the downward spiral can become a positive feedback loop. People who exercise regularly automatically think of it. If they're feeling sluggish, they know exercise will make them feel better. The non-exerciser feels even more sluggish but doesn't have the association that exercise will help.

In the next three sections, I'll review the main benefits of exercise—some well-known and a few that may surprise you. Then I'll discuss the major impediments to exercise in modern society and suggest promising strategies to get moving.

Sitting Ourselves to Death

Statistics about health risks can be dull. The basic message that "Your life depends on it!" can get lost. Physiological researcher Frank Booth, the son of an advertising man, is savvier than most academics about the importance of catchy names. He recently coined the phrase "Sedentary Death Syndrome" and founded "Researchers against Inactivity-related Disorders," or RID, a group of top exercise physiologists who are now lobbying the National Institutes of Health to make exercise a higher priority. RID argues that physical inactivity has an impact on 80–90 percent of the NIH funding areas while presently receiving less than 1 percent of resources.

Booth and his fellow RID researchers advocate an approach that they term "nontraditional" within medical research, but one that is mainstream in evolutionary biology. RID points out that the human genome evolved within an environment of high physical activity. They propose that exercise biologists are not actually studying "the effect of physical activity," but in reality are studying the effect of reintroducing exercise into an unhealthy sedentary population that is genetically programmed for physical activity. "On the basis of healthy gene function, exercise research should thus be viewed from a nontraditional perspective in that the 'control' group should actually be taken from a physically active population," RID argues, "and not from a sedentary population with its predisposition to modern chronic diseases."[6]

Sedentary Death Syndrome hasn't yet caught on as a diagnosis, but its effects are rampant. Approximately 250,000 deaths a year in the United States occur prematurely due to physical inactivity.[7] Many studies that began as examinations of deaths from cardiovascular disease in relation to exercise found that not only these deaths, but also ones from most causes, drop as

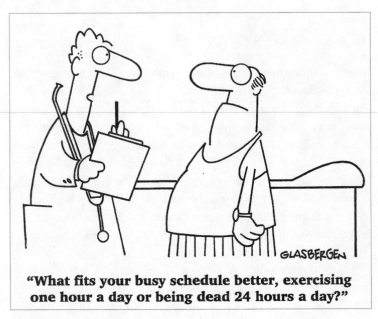

"What fits your busy schedule better, exercising one hour a day or being dead 24 hours a day?"

(Courtesy of Randy Glasbergen, Cartoonist)

exercise levels rise.[8] Most chronic diseases seen in the world today are at least aggravated by inactivity.[9] Specifically heart disease, cancer, diabetes, arthritis and susceptibility to infection have all been linked to lack of exercise.[10] And, of course, obesity is. Estimates of the medical costs of inactivity are now approaching $1 trillion and stand to increase dramatically as the baby boom generation ages.[11]

One study that separated the detrimental effects of inactivity from those of poor eating habits was done with an Old Order Amish community in southern Ontario, Canada. Amish people shun modern conveniences and power machinery. Unlike some other Amish, this Ontario community still farms for a living. Even though they eat what the researchers characterize as a "typical pre–World War II American high-fat, high-sugar

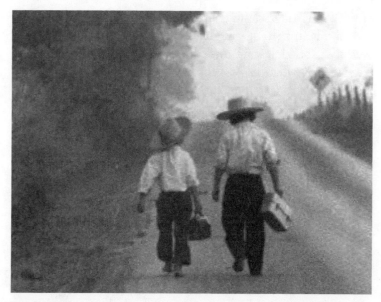

The Old Order Amish shun any technology developed after the mid-1800s. Children walk to school and work in the fields after school (the Amish are exempt from child labor laws). Those lunchboxes likely contain thick cheese sandwiches, cake or other high-starch, high-calorie food, but few Amish are overweight due to their prodigious exercise.

diet"—meat, potatoes, gravy, eggs, garden vegetables, bread, pies and cakes—the Ontario Amish are quite fit. Only 4 percent were obese and only 26 percent were overweight.

Researchers asked ninety-eight of these men and women to wear pedometers (a step-counting device) for seven days. It quickly became evident how they stayed so fit: hard work—and lots of foot power. Their weekly exercise was equivalent to that of runners training for a marathon. Men averaged 18,425 steps a day. Women averaged 14,196.

"The Amish were able to show us just how far we've fallen in the last 150 years or so in terms of the amount of physical activity we typically perform," the lead researcher on the study writes. "Their lifestyle indicates that physical activity played a critical role in keeping our ancestors fit and healthy."[12]

A study of adolescent rats demonstrates how fast the loss of exercise may affect us. Given exercise wheels, adolescent rats grew much stronger than rats without wheels. When experimenters locked the wheels, however, the rats' bodies started to change—quickly. Just five hours after exercise ceased, the rat's abdominal fat cells began emitting chemical signals that made them start to swell. After two days of no exercise, the fat cells got 19 percent larger—and the rats' stomach fat increased by 48 percent.[13]

In a study more relevant to people, it was found that the benefits of exercise start quickly. Over eight months, three-quarters of overweight adults who got even a small amount of exercise—the equivalent of a half hour of brisk walking per day or eleven miles a week—prevented further weight gain. Participants who got no exercise gained an average of 2.5 pounds. Those who did the most vigorous exercise—jogging about seventeen miles weekly—lost an average of nearly eight pounds over eight months *and* lost more than that in fat, on average shedding 10.5 pounds of body fat and gaining 3.5 pounds of lean body mass.[14]

"We eat regularly, and we need to exercise regularly," observes study author David Kump. "There *is* a magic bullet for keeping weight down. It's daily physical activity."[15]

Brain versus Brawn?

Growing up, we all probably heard stereotypes about "dumb jocks" or "muscle brains." When an exercise equipment company mounted an ad campaign featuring muscular athletes with the caption "Body by Nautilus," a popular rejoinder was "Brain by Mattel."

But these clichés have the relationship between fitness and

cognitive abilities backwards. Exercise *improves* alertness, think-ing and memory. The first group of mechanisms through which it does so are ones that benefit the entire body. Exercise stimu-lates the heart and cardiovascular system, improving the circu-lation of blood within the brain. It raises levels of oxygen and other nutrients and aids in the removal of waste products gen-erated by billions of neurons. Longer term, exercise reduces lev-els of artery-clogging cholesterol, preserving blood supply in the brain just as it does elsewhere in the body.

Exercise also has more specific effects on the brain. Scientists once thought that mammalian brains stopped producing cells early in life, but recently it has been discovered that we con-tinue to manufacture new brain cells throughout life. This growth is increased in the face of novel learning situations or social stimulation. However, the most potent stimulant of brain growth is . . . physical exercise.

In *A User's Guide to the Brain*, psychiatrist John Ratey refers to exercise as "Miracle-Gro."[16] Exercise increases levels of brain-derived neurotrophic factor (BDNF).[17] BDNF both stimulates the production of new brain cells—neurons—and promotes their survival.[18] Exercise especially generates neurons in the hippocampus, an organ associated with memory, and these new neurons have been demonstrated to enhance learning.[19] Addi-tionally, exercise raises levels of the neurotransmitters dopamine and norepinephrine which facilitate attention and concentration and help "lock in" memories when they form.

At all ages, physical activity seems to improve learning and thinking. A 2002 California Department of Education study reported that the more physical education classes students took, the higher their level of academic achievement.[20] A large, five-year study recently found that physical activity in later years was associated with lower risks of cognitive impairment, Alzheimer's disease and dementia in general.[21] Another concluded that if exercise began by early middle age, it reduced the risk of developing Alzheimer's even further.[22] These data from humans are supported by animal research demonstrating that exercise can increase neuronal survival and resilience to brain trauma,[23] and promote the growth of new blood vessels in the brain.[24] The sea squirt is not just an amusing metaphor, but an extreme example of an under-recognized principle: brains exist largely to coordinate movement, and they require movement to function well.

Combating Depression with Exercise

Several recent studies report the "new finding" that exercise is an effective treatment for depression. Actually, this has been known for decades. Thirty years ago, two studies had already established that running and other exercise programs were effective treatments for depression.[25] Twenty years ago, running had been shown to help depression as much as the class of antidepressants then most widely prescribed, the tricyclics.[26] A recent study reproduced this effect, comparing the use of stationary bikes and treadmills to Zoloft, one of the new serotonin-reuptake inhibitors—the class into which Prozac falls.[27] One hundred and fifty patients diagnosed with depression followed one of three treatment programs: exercise, Zoloft or both. At the end of the four-month study, all three groups displayed significantly lower depression rates. Six-month follow-up examinations revealed that subjects in the exercise group experienced lower relapse rates than those given the Zoloft or combination treatments. Reviews of the various studies of exercise for depression have concluded that exercise is effective both short and long term[28] and that aerobic activity, strength training and flexibility training all prove effective in treating depression.[29]

It has long been a mystery why all antidepressant drugs take ten days to three weeks to work despite the fact that the chemicals reach therapeutic levels in the bloodstream and brain within hours. Their initial known effect is on a variety of neurotransmitters. The serotonin-reuptake inhibitors act on serotonin, while other drugs affect dopamine or norepinephrine. They raise the level of these different neurotransmitters rapidly—and yet they all show the same time lag for a therapeutic effect. Electroshock treatments, when they alleviate depression, show a similar delay. One of the newest theories about the cause and treatment of depression offers an explanation of the delay. This theory postulates that depression occurs when there is a deficit of neurons being produced in the brain, and that antidepressants work by stimulating neurogenesis—the same mechanism I've just discussed by which exercise enhances learning and thinking. Modern brain-imaging studies indeed report that long-term depressed patients have fewer neurons in the hippocampus. All known treatments for depression, from drugs to electroshock to exercise, have been found to stimulate neurogenesis. It turns out that the lag-time in improvement from depression is about the time that it takes the newly generated neurons to mature and begin to function.

Exercise does other things that affect depression. Beta-endorphins—milder natural cousins of morphine and heroin—are produced by exercise. These are the cause of the short-term "runner's high," though they may have little to do with the longer-term improvement in mood.[30] Besides creating new neurons, physical activity enhances other forms of neuroplasticity—the ability of the brain to change. Exercise stimulates serotonin, along with the catecholamines that aid memory storage and may also raise mood.[31] Exercise has also been found to benefit other psychological problems, including anxiety and insomnia. It makes people more resilient to psychological stress, probably because it helps to regulate the stress hormone cortisol. Both aerobic and strength-building exercise seem to have similar beneficial effects.

As Suburbs Grow Larger, So Do Suburbanites

We often think of suburbs as healthier than cities: grass, trees, fresh air—right? Certainly the air is not as polluted. But city life, no matter how unnatural in other ways, does involve more walking. Average suburban dwellers walk less than half as much as their city cousins.

A 2003 special issue of the journal *Public Health* published several studies reporting that suburbanites are heavier than city dwellers and have higher rates of many weight-related health problems. This was true even once researchers statistically controlled for other factors such as race, age and economic status. One study focused on obesity, finding that people in the most sprawling suburban areas weigh six pounds more than people in more densely developed cityscapes. Another survey found that suburbanites reported more chronic health problems, including high blood pressure, arthritis, headaches, migraines and breathing problems, than people who lived in cities.[32] The worst possible place to call home, this study reported, was what's often the American ideal: a cul-de-sac with few sidewalks that empties into a big access road so that residents drive to shop or to go to school and work.

Another article in the special issue found that among large cities, the most densely populated ones had thinner and healthier residents than the more sparsely populated ones—again controlling for race, age and income. These healthier cities were the most suitable for walking—Boston, Chicago, New York, San Francisco and Seattle. The cities with the lowest population density and the least ease of walking—Atlanta, Houston and Phoenix—had the highest rates of diabetes and obesity. The average adult in a sprawling city such as Atlanta had the health characteristics of someone four years older in a more compact city like Seattle.[33]

"We do an environmental impact statement for a new subdivision, and we look at trees and birds and the rest," commented Dr. Richard Jackson, the director of the National Center for Environmental Health and editor of the special issue. "But we need to look at the impacts on human health.[34]

America's most densely populated city, New York, has examined variations within its own boroughs—all densely populated by other cities' standards. The highest density of all, of course, is Manhattan. Manhattanites are trim compared to national standards. The extent of the difference is partially masked by the fact that it has a large population of minorities who tend to be heavier for a variety of economic, dietary and lifestyle reasons. When city researchers analyzed the data for white Manhattan residents, only 34 percent were overweight, compared with 64 percent of whites elsewhere in America. And just 7 percent of white Manhattan residents were obese—one-third the national rate of 21 percent.[35] "The proportion of whites in Manhattan who are not obese is striking," says Dr. Thomas Frieden, the city's health commissioner. "I wish we could find out the reason why and bottle it."[36]

We do of course know much of the reason: walking, climbing stairs, walking, bicycling, walking. Patterns overseas are similar. Shanghai and Beijing, where people walk and ride bicycles, have relatively thin populations. However, those cities' new suburbs, where people drive more, are developing high rates of diabetes and obesity.[37]

Critics of the conclusions in the *Public Health* studies argue that the research correlations don't prove suburban living causes the higher weight and health problems. They maintain that the cause could go in the other direction: that heavier people and those with health problems find walking more difficult and leave the city for settings where they can drive everywhere.

The cause may well go both ways, but there's pressure to be less active once you live in the suburbs. A friend of mine recently moved to the idyllic suburb of Newton, Massachusetts, with great public schools—one near enough that he assumed his children could recreate his childhood ritual of walking to school. But not only has the prevalence of sidewalks changed, so has behavior. My friend found that few parents let their kids walk to school, because it is considered more dangerous than a generation ago (it's not clear that it actually is). So he didn't send his children off as his parents had, but walked with them the brief route to school. Other parents constantly stopped to offer rides, assuming his car must be in the shop—why else would anybody walk? When parents got to the school driveway, they'd wait and maneuver to drop off their children as few feet from the school door as possible. It's hard to go against the local customs.

Ghosts of Environments Past

If the suburbs are bad for people, why do so many of us flock there? The explanation, as usual, lies in our instincts, which don't urge us strongly to exercise but do tell us what kind of environment should be safe and nurturing—or rather, which ones would have been for hunter-gatherers ten thousand years ago.

Humans evolved on the African savannah—flat grasslands with a few scattered trees and bushes. There were some hills with sparser food and some forests with more predators, so humans stuck to the open grassy areas when they could. Camping by a pond or stream was obviously a plus.

Researchers find that when they show pictures of landscapes to people anywhere in the world, the favorite scene is the same: flat, lush green grass, a few trees but no forests unless they're in the background, fresh water nearby.[38] Personal experience plays some role—people raised amid ice-peaked mountains are likelier to rate these higher than the desert and vice versa. However, landscapes that recreate the primeval savannah are given much higher marks than simple personal exposure would predict. Around the planet, people who can afford it go to great expense importing lawn grass into areas that are naturally rocky hills, dense forest or sandy desert. They irrigate and fertilize these transplanted lawns. A major health danger in suburbia is the amount of fertilizer and pesticide poured into making yards *look* healthy.[39]

None of America's fifty varieties of grass planted in yards is indigenous to our continent. The grasses that herds of deer, antelope and buffalo grazed on before the European settlers arrived were sparser and less intensely green. Early in America's history, settlers imported grass that mimicked the savannah— they were already cultivating it in Europe. In the north, we grow varieties that will keep more chlorophyll during their dormant winter phase, and everywhere grass is chemically prodded to keep it green. The desperate fight not to let one's yard go brown in winter seems to be related to the common aversion to bare, leafless winter trees—in the warmer savannah these would have denoted plant death. Elsewhere in the world, different strains of lawn grass have been adapted to keep yards in the Middle East and Scandinavia resembling savannah.

The most affluent people can mimic the rarer but yet more desirable position of camping near a water source by purchasing property with a pond or stream—or putting in a swimming pool with a bottom painted aqua blue to simulate especially clean water. Bird-feeders attract potential game. Even the much-maligned plastic lawn flamingo—the butt of jokes while selling 450,000 per year—likely owes its popularity to recreating the long-legged birds of the savannah.

Once the illusion is complete, do we go out and exercise in it? Of course not. If camp was stocked with food, no sensible hunter-gatherer would have ventured forth to search for more. Instead, we set our thermostats to 72 degrees—the average temperature of the savannah—and enjoy our green grassy views from behind glass.

Our little backyard pseudo-savannahs are yet another example of supernormal stimuli. Ironically, the less natural-looking city environment holds more cues and opportunities to keep us moving in a natural manner. When the *New York Times* reported the study on health in different areas, it quoted a former Manhattanite who'd moved to the suburbs and found herself not even walking the half-mile, ten-minute walk to her commuter train station. "It's next to the South Mountain Reservation," she said. "It's all woods and dark, and you feel like you're in *The Blair Witch Project*. So there goes the walking."[40]

It's very unlikely that a path beside a wooded reservoir is really more dangerous than the city street she walked along before. Evolution has led us to weigh some risks more heavily

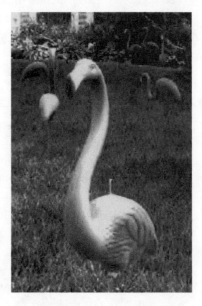

The Lawn Flamingo: In 1952, the Union Plastics Company of Massachusetts introduced the first flamingo lawn ornament. It was a crude Styrofoam cutout and dogs loved to chew it up. Four years later, the company hired twenty-one-year-old art student Don Featherstone (real name!) to sculpt the more lifelike hard plastic version we see today. Featherstone's design is based on the American pink flamingo, but it's very similar to the African flamingos of the primeval savannahs. The much-ridiculed decoration sells 450,000 copies a year. *(Courtesy of Katie Inlow, Stork Greetings & More Lawn Displays, www.storkgreetings.com)*

than they merit in the twenty-first century. Studies show that we enormously overestimate risks from both rare and violent events and underrate the risks of the common but mundane—car accidents, cancer, diabetes. Most of us really don't think about the latter unless they're happening to someone we know. Violent events are easy to imagine; we have instincts to worry about attacks from enemies and, as the quote above demonstrates, horror movies to reinforce them. Neither one features images of a gradual decline from diabetes.

Spectator Nation

There were, of course, instincts that got our ancestors moving: ones to hunt, explore, practice skills—and fight. Conflict used to occur both as bitter battles between enemies and as controlled jostling for dominance within a group. These urges are not utilized for most of us now that food is already gathered and work tasks are sedentary. In modern times, when there isn't a war or natural disaster in progress, these impulses have their main outlet in sports. Games range from simple catch and tag among children to elaborate competitions between the most athletic young men of the community.

Those playing get some exercise—though as we'll see in a minute, team sports are generally not the optimal activity. Some sports have always been dangerous: the losers in the Roman Coliseum often died; three out of four professional boxers have some detectable brain damage.[41] But the biggest problem with most sports is that they quickly become spectator events—the impetus to move is channeled into vicarious experience for the spectators.

Until recently, many games had a ratio of players to spectators of between 1:1 and 1:3. The viewers often moved around

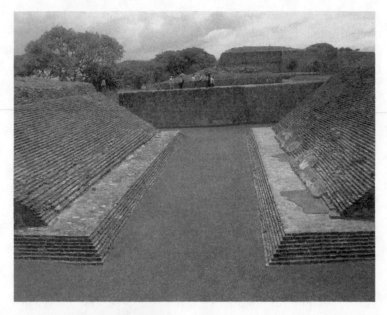

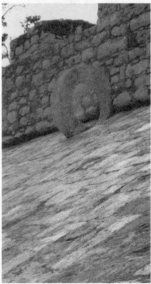

Mayan basketball: For 3,500 years, beginning shortly after the Central American
hunter-gatherers settled down and started
farming, Olmecs, Toltecs, Aztecs and
Mayans played a ballgame that was sort of
a cross between soccer and basketball.
Players would bounce a rubber ball up and
down a walled court, shaped like a capital
I, trying to pass the ball through a serpent-
inscribed stone hoop twenty feet above
the ground. At some point in the game's
history, the rules included beheading the
captain of the losing team. Spectators
stood atop the walls and on the steps of
temples at either end of the court.
(Left: photo courtesy of Ian Ruderman.
Above: photo courtesy of the author)

the perimeter to get a better view of the action. And they walked to get to the arena. The modern version subverts the "gaming instinct" further from exercise. Crowds drive to huge stadiums serving beer and hot dogs. Or spectators simply sit in home recliners using the remote to switch between two games while chowing down on delivered pizza.

Even aside from the inert spectators, exercise for players is often limited. In reading how unfit suburbanites are, it may have occurred to the reader that this is exactly where sports—at least for children—are supposed to flourish. "Little League Dad" and "Soccer Mom" are suburban stereotypes. But much of these activities involves purchasing uniforms and suiting up to drive to a game that may be in another suburb on the far side of the city—where the parent hopes the coach will let their child play rather than sit on the sidelines. It takes a major commitment of time from parent and child but, as the researcher of the urban/suburban study notes, "During those thirty minutes that they actually play soccer each week," he said, "they may not spend even half the amount of energy that another kid spends walking to school."[42]

What happened to throwing a ball or Frisbee around on that trophy lawn? Certainly there are other skills, such as social ones, to be gained from team sports—but these would also be learned by kids working out disagreements that occur as they throw a Frisbee around their backyard.

One reason that both after-hours programs and school's dwindling physical education hours are spent teaching rules for various games is the rationale that they're setting people up with skills for exercise across their lifespan. However, research shows that less than 5 percent of the population older than twenty-four uses team sports as a form of physical activity.[43] It's time to think of new approaches, and a few programs are doing that.

No Child Left on Their Behind

"When I taught physical education and team sports, it was by the book," recalls Phil Lawler, director of the PE4life Institute and physical education coordinator for School District 203 in Naperville, Illinois. Class lasted forty-two minutes. "When kids went to PE, we would take attendance; then teams were picked. The team put on tennis shoes and got on the field, gathered into a huddle, called a play, and went to the line of scrimmage. The best athlete was quarterback and his best friend receiver. When play began, fifteen to twenty kids were standing around, doing nothing. We spent a lot of time arguing about who was offside and about conflict management."

Lawler and the PE instructors working for him analyzed the forty-two-minute period to discover just how many kids were truly moving in class and physically active—how many kids actually touched the ball. "Something was wrong with this picture. We threw out the whole concept of teaching sports."[44]

In the early 1990s, Lawler redesigned the PE curriculum for Naperville so that it would actually educate students about exercise and health and improve their fitness levels. He wanted a program that could be enjoyable for all students, not just those who were gifted athletes. Imagine a classroom in which only the most gifted students are allowed to speak, and the rest are only spectators!

Lawler raised money for hi-tech cardiovascular equipment—heart monitors, treadmills, rowing machines, steppers—to maximize individual movement and effort for every student. With heart monitors to measure resting heart rate after cardiovascular workouts, students got credit for their personal efforts instead of comparisons with the more adept athletes. The initial program emphasized cardiovascular training, but as research emerged through the late 1990s that strength training was just as important, Lawler added weight training.

Naperville students take daily physical education from sixth grade through high school. Some classes are required of everyone, including fitness, dance, aquatics and gymnastics. Students can choose among electives including a high ropes course, rock-climbing and kayaking in the pool. Team sports are still an option but in a form that keeps everyone moving: football is four on four with no line of scrimmage, basketball two on two. Students exercise in T-shirts emblazoned with "Naperville

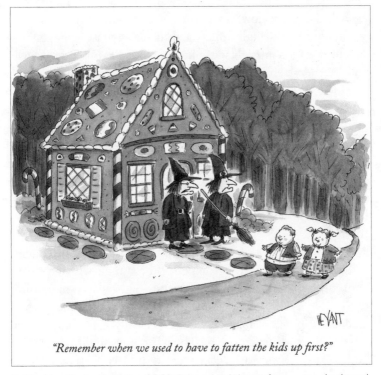

"Remember when we used to have to fatten the kids up first?"

Physical Education" on their front and "The Surgeon General has determined that an inactive lifestyle can be detrimental to your health" on their sleeves.

Lawler's department gives an initial fitness test to every child to establish a baseline. The first time the tests were administered, the results were scary. Only 22 percent were in the "heart-healthy" range—able to run a mile in seven and a half to ten minutes. After a decade of the new PE, students are now fitter than their contemporaries at other schools and their predecessors. In a comparison with a school in California with very similar demographics, 33 percent of the California high school freshmen are overweight or obese; out of Naperville's 19,000 students, only 3 percent are overweight or obese.[45] Eighty percent of them can now run in the "heart-healthy" zone. Ninety-seven percent now fall into a healthy fat-to-muscle range.[46]

The CDC named Naperville a model PE program. Lawler caught the attention of the newly formed national nonprofit PE4life and was appointed its director. Their Naperville offices now offer seminars for heath personnel and PE teachers from around the nation—with observational visits to the Naperville schools. Representatives from the American Cancer Society and the American Heart Association recently attended the seminars. "I told them that we need their clout more than we need their money," Lawler says. "The general population just hasn't made the shift yet to preventive measures when it comes to health."[47]

One of the reasons cited by other school systems for reducing or eliminating PE is the competition for time with academic content, or with preparation for the high-stakes standardized exams. Naperville's experience proves that this attitude is misguided. In 1999, several years into the new PE curriculum, Naperville's eighth graders took the Third International Mathematics and Science Study (TIMSS) test along with students from thirty-eight other nations. The Naperville students ranked first in science for the entire world and sixth in math—scoring number one in the United States for this also.[48]

Naperville is an affluent town located near Bell Laboratories. Seventy-one percent of Naperville parents have college degrees—far above national norms. No one, not even Lawler, would suggest that the schools owe their spectacular scores solely to their PE program. But it obviously didn't hurt academics and probably helped, consistent with the California study correlating hours of PE with academic achievement and with general findings about the effects of exercise on the brain.

Lawler is sometimes criticized by fans of old-fashioned team sports for taking the competitive edge away from his physical education program. "My response to that," he says, "is: 'Take on the challenge of managing your own health, weight, blood pressure and cholesterol. Where are you in *that* competition?' Most Americans are not winning."[49]

How to Start Winning at Fitness

There are three basic strategies people in our society can take to get a decent amount of exercise: 1) modern gym or home fitness equipment engineered to mimic what we used to do naturally; 2) rediscovering one's favorite sport(s); and 3) considering a job that builds in exercise. Each has its merits.

Gyms. They're the standard middle-class solution to the dilemma and the most practical one for lifelong non-exercisers—which makes them my personal choice.

Unlike natural athletes, whom I'll discuss in a minute, I enjoyed a bookwormish youth. I got some exercise—my generation played outside, walked all over large campuses and danced at parties. But when anyone suggested vigorous athletics, I'm embarrassed at how often I quoted W. C. Fields: "When I feel the urge to exercise, I lie down until it passes." Any photo of

Fields should have told me it was his wit, not his health habits, I wanted to emulate.

Fortunately I took to heart the sixties' and seventies' enthusiasm for "health food," so, with the forgiving metabolism of youth, I was slim and energetic without much exercise. In my early thirties, I began sitting at a desk more and driving to get places, and my metabolism would have been slowing down in any case. I found pounds creeping on and my energy diminishing. I looked around to see what my healthiest friends were doing. For the most part it was running—or rather "jogging," as the craze was called then. This is one of the simplest and best forms of exercise, but I had bad shoes or jumped into it too aggressively, so my initial attempts yielded more joint pain than exercise. I didn't persist long enough to get it right because a newer phenomenon proved a better fit for me.

The health club—the exercise gym renamed and retooled for the average non-athlete. By then, every town had one. Now they're every few blocks. There are gyms or "health clubs" or "fitness centers" for every budget, from designer-decorated saunas to local YMCA fitness rooms or high school gyms charging nominal fees to the community during off hours. Gyms are friendly. The only tales I've heard of ones where only young people who look great in spandex are welcome or where you'll get laughed out if you can't bench-press your own weight are from people who hadn't actually visited the establishment in question but somehow "just knew" this.

My present gym in Cambridge, Massachusetts, is the least expensive option after the local Y and high school. It's a windowless warehouse filled with an array of exercise equipment and a mix of Harvard faculty, ethnic populations, students, senior citizens, serious athletes and cardiac patients. These groups interact more amiably than they do in some other settings. Even when I briefly belonged to a gym frequented by competitive bodybuilders and overheard alarming conversations about illegal steroids, I was still struck that these same guys were quick to offer their spot on a machine to a pregnant woman or to help an elderly man struggling to figure out a piece of equipment. I've always found people are really, really nice at gyms—the opposite of the stereotype of spectators at sports events, where even Little League parents can get nasty. And this makes sense. Research finds that building up adrenaline and related excitement hormones intended to enable quicker action creates stress and irritability when one doesn't get to move. On the other hand, as we've discussed, actually exercising has very positive effects on mood.

Health clubs have come to realize that collectively they've enrolled most of the athletically inclined. Instead of competing with each other for this minority of America, they are now reaching out to the great inert majority. Half of their initiatives are commendable—ads show more people of all sizes and ages exercising. They're trying to let the out-of-shape know they're welcome, that they don't have to look like models before coming in. The other half of the initiatives are alarming—the equivalent of the new junk foods with "Lite" or "Natural" labeling chunks of fats and sugars. "We don't want them to be put off by weights clanking," and "People grunting or sweating tend to scare them," remark two marketing consultants as they describe promotions emphasizing lounge chairs, snacks, soothing music and "gentle stretching."[50] These ads cater to the well-founded hope that people will pay to feel as if they're exercising when they're not.

So beware of gyms trying to collude with you to pretend you're exercising when you're not. Stretching and relaxation are beneficial, but don't let anyone tell you they substitute for exercise. If you're *really* in need of the gentlest start because of injuries or arthritis, you probably want to go to a physical therapist; your doctor may refer you and your insurance may pay. Otherwise, you want a serious gym with clanking weights.

In picking one, you want to decide what facilities you'll use.

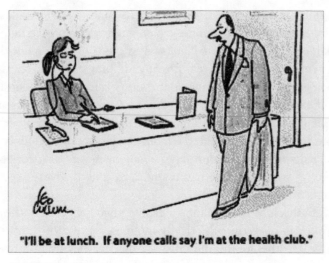

"I'll be at lunch. If anyone calls say I'm at the health club."

(© 2007 Leo Cullum from cartoonbank.com)

If you're quite social, then you may want the largest selection of classes—both strength training and aerobic. "Classes" is somewhat of a misnomer because, though most do teach you something the first few times, they largely just give you a set time to show up, a cheerleader up front urging you to challenge yourself and a set-up that guarantees you won't quit in the middle unless you're genuinely exhausted.

If you're more independent and have good self-discipline, then you may want to look for the gym with the most weight equipment and cardio machines (treadmills, stair-climbers, ski-tracks, rowing machines). For strength training, if you're a beginner, the weight machines make it harder to do something wrong; but with more experience, free weights may give you the best workout. It's a good idea to hire a personal trainer for the first few sessions to show you what to do on the machines if the gym doesn't provide this service automatically for new members. I know people who pay a trainer for every workout three to five times a week, but this is hardly cost-effective for anyone not training for the Olympics. If you're short on self-discipline but don't want to do classes, consider joining with a friend who'll coordinate workouts. And home gym equipment is best for those for whom time constraints are the biggest issue—but you'd better be high on the self-discipline continuum.

Whatever approach you choose, make sure it fits your style. Gym regulars watch the New Year's resolution crowd fill classes and occupy machines for a couple of weeks each year, disappearing by the third week of January. Though owners and regulars delight in the fact that these people subsidize the gym (often with full-year memberships) while not taking up space, you don't want to fall into this group.

Sports. Does the thought of a ball field, tennis court or swimming pool fill you with nostalgia? If you loved one or more sports in your youth, that's a gift that makes it easier to return to exercise. The drawback of gyms and classes is that they're so routine and repetitive; many people find them dull, and you have to get your reinforcement from noticing that you feel better. Sports, for their devotees, don't feel arbitrary; some hunter-gatherer instinct that's really intended for finding food and shelter or for defeating an enemy gets channeled toward hitting a ball, getting a ball through a hoop or reaching the end of a track first. We just need to unhook these impulses from spectator sports and reconnect them with real movement.

Many adults who drifted away from an early athletic start believe they can't play unless they're young again or unless they're better than they ever were. But once you give up those self-imposed limits, it's easier than ever to play sports at any level. There are beginner leagues and age-ranked competitions for most every game. In a few sports, it's better to modify them a bit for later life. If you played tackle football, decades later touch football is a wiser choice. Perhaps consider softball instead of baseball this time round. But many sports—swimming, cycling,

tennis and racketball—serve their players well into late life.
Dance, not usually classified as a sport, is similarly rewarding for
those who re-engage with it—and again, once you get over the
idea that you have to be great at it, there are many welcoming
venues.

Martial arts and ballet present a mental challenge, requiring all
one's concentration to coordinate movements. Team sports, part-
nered games and ballroom dance engage social skills. But sports
characterized by repetitiveness and solitude also have advantages
for some people. When I interviewed people for an earlier book
on creativity in dreaming, I was struck by how often low dream-
recallers who hadn't had breakthrough dreams told me that their
"aha!" inspirations came during repetitive exercise—swimming
laps, running at a moderate pace, or cycling at steady speed
through familiar territory. Research shows that people perform
intellectual tasks best in the hour right after exercise, so company
softball teams and lunchtime jogs are good for productivity. If
your workplace doesn't have what you want, organize it.

Work. The final answer to the modern dilemma is to arrange
a job that involves exercise. This is the most natural solution—
our Stone Age ancestors got their exercise during the daily tasks
of living. Today, most people think of work as inherently a desk
job. But there are likely to be alternatives. The standard advice
is: park further away from your office door, use the stairs instead
of the elevator. These are sound recommendations, but they're
only a start. If you're going to get most of your exercise on the
job, you want to think of major changes.

Since I'm a psychologist, many of the examples I know of come
from my own field. Though I get my exercise in my spare time, a
number of colleagues have arranged careers that involve exercise.
One of my friends does psychotherapy with adolescents—an age
range for whom it's common advice that going for a walk during
the session makes it easier to talk than sitting opposite each other
in chairs. My friend has taken this a step further and decided

that walking is the default option for his sessions and that sitting in chairs for an hour is the alternative offered if a teen objects. Since I do a lot of hypnotherapy in which patients need to relax and close their eyes, I've walked only with weight-loss patients and only with those not undergoing hypnotherapy. I've offered the mobile session to some and virtually insisted on it with others who were procrastinating about beginning exercise on their own. It didn't interfere with conversation in the way I had anticipated—though Cambridge is unusual in that, unlike rural settings, it does have sidewalks, yet unlike cities those sidewalks are uncrowded and conversations feel private. In the heyday of psychoanalysis, leaving the office would have been frowned upon, but now cognitive-behavioral therapists often walk with clients over bridges and onto elevators when desensitizing them to phobias.

It is possible to walk while having a business discussion in most professional fields. Two-person meetings take place in offices even on nice days and when no equipment is needed, partly because no one thinks to suggest, "How about we go for a walk while we talk about this?" And, as everyone knows, you can certainly make your phone calls while walking around.

Three other psychologists I know have retooled their practices more radically. They all worked in health psychology or behavior medicine and had grown tired of sitting and/or grown frustrated with the limits of talk therapy for physical problems. All three got certified as fitness trainers. One pursues the two careers separately, booking psychotherapy and exercise clients into different blocks of time at the office or gym respectively. The other two have combined the roles, so they may have the first session with a client in the office and later ones at the gym while working on cognitive-behavioral interventions on weight loss, cardiac rehabilitation or sports psychology.

Professionals in any field can find a way to exercise as they work. A biologist friend of mine, Mark Moffett, never fancied a career sitting over lab specimens or around a seminar table. From the minute his graduate classes included field work, Mark was off spelunking through dark tunnels in search of blind cave tarantulas, climbing the world's tallest tree and hiking around the Kalahari with the !Kung. Another friend, physician Ken Kamler, is a hand surgeon the half of the year he's practicing conventional medicine. However, he's also developed a specialty in extreme emergency medicine that allows him to indulge his love of climbing as the physician on many Everest ascents and a medical researcher on deep-sea dives. Two schoolteachers I've known grew tired of the classroom and used their credentials to work in wilderness learning centers where students rotate through for a week of outdoor exploration. But the vast majority of physicians, biologists and schoolteachers think of themselves as being in inherently sedentary jobs—and ones so time-consuming that they have trouble getting any exercise.

Less skilled jobs also have equivalents which are healthier. Entry-level construction jobs tend to pay higher salaries than entry-level assembly line work or store clerking. Some demand heavy lifting, but many do not. Assistants to electricians and plumbers carry modest loads around and fetch tools. If your main job experience is working a cash register, why sit on a stool at a convenience store reaching up to get the occasional pack of cigarettes for a customer when the same job at a local garden center would include frequent walks around the lot carrying plants back to the payment desk? For every nightwatchman's position in front of a bank of video monitors, there's one patrolling the grounds on foot.

One of the most dramatic shifts to a physically challenging job that I've seen was by my friend Susan. Susan didn't undertake her change for the health benefits. She was at least forty pounds overweight and getting virtually no exercise—I'd been alarmed when we attended an artists' "open studios" and she got winded climbing a single flight of stairs. Susan's job was about to end, as it was funded by a two-year federal grant to work with families of 9/11 victims (because two of the planes had taken off from Logan airport, Boston suffered the third most deaths after New York and Washington, D.C). Susan was depressed and was not immediately landing another position in the tight Boston job market. Determined to continue trauma counseling, she found an opening in an African refugee camp working with torture survivors from the Liberian civil war. The job started immediately, and Susan left Boston to the amazement of her friends. For a year, we got occasional emails from the communal Internet connection, tales about counseling the traumatized that in many ways seemed universal interspersed with details unique to her refugee camp: group therapy interrupted by snakes crawling into the hut, a spider bite that left Susan's eye swollen shut for two days. At the end of a year, she came through Boston for a few days—she was taking another job in Sierra Leone supporting witnesses for the UN's special war crimes tribunal. For other purposes, the story would be one of the triumph of the human spirit in the face of atrocities. But for the topic of the present book, the superficial things are most relevant: when I saw Susan after a year, she was thirty-five pounds lighter with great muscle tone and radiated energy and vitality. Certainly the experience of palpably helping those in need every day contributed to her transformation. But Susan attributed much of it also to the lifestyle. The American, European and African staff lived in conditions only a bit better than those of the refugees. They often ate only supper—small meals of roasted chicken and bulgur. Fruit was the only food in plentiful supply. They carried their own water in buckets and walked everywhere they went within the sprawling camp. The main form of recreation was dancing to Congolese music at night.

Career changes that increase exercise can benefit people at any point on the fitness continuum. My schoolteacher friend who went to work for the outdoor children's camp went from fairly fit to super-fit over the first year. One advantage of the most radical changes is that they're often self-perpetuating. If you take a job in the middle of Africa or an American mountain range, you're not going to have to decide anew each day whether you're going to exercise—it will just happen. Though most people are well aware of the sacrifices involved in radical lifestyle changes, they're out of touch with some of the wonderful benefits of making the change and also with the sacrifices in lost years of life and health that just continuing their sedentary ways incurs. In Chapters 8 and 9, I'll talk more about how you can motivate yourself and others to make changes large and small. In the next chapter we'll examine one of the major enemies of exercise in our culture—television.

5

Thinking Outside the Box

"*Boob tube*," "idiot box," "one-eyed monster." Nicknames for television betray our concern even as we try to laugh it off. Just as people cheerfully admit to being "couch potatoes" who eat "junk food" with no intention of exercising or eating better, "TV addicts" who are "glued to the tube" rarely try to wean themselves from the "glass tit." Fifteen years ago, researchers posed a question to children of intact families: if they had to give up either their father or their television set for one week, which would go? Care to guess how they answered? I'll tell you at the end of the chapter.

In the article "Television Addiction," psychologists Robert Kubey and Mihaly Csikszentmihalyi observe, "Perhaps the most ironic aspect of the struggle for survival is how easily organisms can be harmed by that which they desire. The trout is caught by the fisherman's lure, the mouse by cheese. But at least those creatures have the excuse that bait and cheese look like sustenance. Humans seldom have that consolation."[1]

Animals and man are indeed often harmed by what they desire—especially when encountering new stimuli for which evolution hasn't prepared them. That's the central thesis of this book. But I believe that the human television viewer has very much the same "consolation," "excuse" or explanation as the fish on the hook. The trout lure mimics—or exceeds—the darting and bright coloration of the tastiest fly; television mimics—or exceeds—the adventures, athletics and human connections that we desire but actually miss out on as we stare at a box of electric circuitry. Television is another instance of the supernormal stimulus—in this case masquerading as activity rather than food.

Adults in the industrial world average three hours a day of television viewing—half their leisure time and more than any other single activity besides work or sleep. Children and adolescents watch more yet. "By the time most Americans are eighteen years old, they have spent more time in front of the television set than they have spent in school, and far more than they have spent talking with their teachers, their friends or even their parents," observes Newton Minow, former chairman of the FCC. In the course of a lifetime, the average American will have logged nine solid years in front of the television.

Remember the most common reason people cite for not exercising? The most common reason for eating junk food instead of preparing healthy meals?

How does television steal so much time? Though there's much to decry about its content—and we'll get to that shortly—the most sinister aspect of television lies in the medium itself. There's a growing body of research on what it does to our brains—"idiot box" is not far off.

Humans have a basic instinct to pay attention to any sudden or novel stimulus, usually a movement or sound. In 1927, the legendary Russian neurologist Ivan Pavlov named this reflex the "orienting response." The orienting response, shared with other animals, is part of our evolutionary heritage. It evolved to spot and assess game, potential mates, enemies or predators. The orienting person or animal turns eyes and ears in the direction of the stimulus and then freezes while parts of the brain associated with new learning become more active. Blood vessels to the brain dilate, those to muscles constrict, the heart slows and alpha waves—the brain's slower, relaxed rhythms—are blocked for a few seconds.

By the age of six months, babies orient when a television is turned on. Adults continue to do so. Even researchers studying the effect are not immune: "Among life's more embarrassing moments have been countless occasions when I am engaged in conversation in a room while a TV set is on, and I cannot for the life of me stop from periodically glancing over to the screen," confesses Percy Tannenbaum of the University of California, Berkeley. "This occurs not only during dull conversations but during reasonably interesting ones just as well."[2]

Psychologists have found that the formal features of television—cuts, zooms, pans and sudden noises—all activate the orienting response.[3] More recent research shows that the effect persists initially for four to six seconds after each stimulus. Producers of educational television for children have found that judicious orchestration of these formal features can increase learning—presumably by keeping children focused on the screen. After a certain level of intensity, however, the orienting response is overworked and reverse effects on learning and attention begin. This is what is seen with commercials, action sequences and music videos, where formal features provoke orienting at the rapid-fire rate of one per second. After a few minutes of this bombardment, one sees a strange mix of physiological signs of high and low attention. Eyes stay focused, the body is still and directed toward the set, but learning and memory drop to lower levels than when not orienting. Measurements of metabolism (including calorie-burning) average 14.5 percent *lower* when watching television than when simply lying in bed.[4] EEG studies similarly find less mental stimulation, as measured by alpha brainwaves, during viewing than during reading or other quiet activities.

When researchers query people watching television, most viewers report feeling relaxed but passive and not alert—in keeping with their physiological signs. The minute the set is turned off, the relaxation ends, but the passivity and lowered alertness continue. Many feel as if television has somehow sucked out all their energy. People say they have more trouble concentrating after viewing than before. In contrast, few indicate such problems after reading. After playing sports or engaging in hobbies, people report improvements in mood. After watching television, most people's moods are either about the same or worse than before.[5]

These are the short-term negative effects, but what about the long term? An article in *Pediatrics* reported that the longer chil-

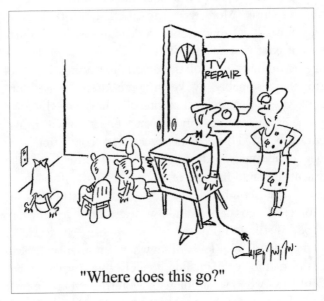

"Where does this go?"

(Courtesy of www.CartoonStock.com)

dren sit in front of a television, the less likely they are to sleep well.[6] Children who view more television are likelier to have behavioral problems, including attention deficit hyperactivity disorder (ADHD), and to perform worse academically. In a study of 1,797 children, Frederick Zimmerman found that watching television before the age of three was linked to poorer reading and math skills at the ages of six and seven. "For those who watch more than three hours of television per day before age three, the negative impact is similar to the adverse effect of large differences in maternal IQ or education," Zimmerman wrote.[7] In a study of 2,000 children, for every hour per day watched at age one and age three, the children had a 10 percent higher chance of developing diagnosed ADHD by age seven. A toddler watching three hours of infant television daily therefore had a 30 percent higher chance of ADHD. A British study found that children exposed to the most television before the age of two were delayed in talking.[8] "In question is whether the insistent noise of television in the home may interfere with the development of 'inner speech' by which a child learns to think through problems and plans," wrote child brain expert Jane Healy, in discussing these findings.[9]

Adults who watch more television also report a higher rate of mood and intellectual difficulties. The television industry argues that this doesn't prove causation: people with these problems might then be inclined toward excessive viewing. However, one study, now two decades old, seems to demonstrate direct causation between television and many of these difficulties. In the 1980s, researchers at the University of British Columbia got a unique opportunity when several remote Canadian mountain communities, which had never had broadcast television, contracted to receive it by cable. The researchers surveyed people's activities and tested them on a variety of cognitive and behavioral measures before television was installed and for five years after. Immediately, the number of hours devoted to sports declined, along with dancing and all other physically active leisure pursuits. Over time, both adults and children in the town became less creative on problem-solving tests, less able to persevere at tasks and less tolerant of unstructured time.

And Now a Word from Our Sponsor

The passive, hands-free daze of television is an obvious time to consume junk food, and advertisers make sure viewers receive a constant bombardment of suggestions to do so. With their average of three hours of television a day, Americans get 22,000 commercials a year, 5,000 of them for food products—mostly for low-nutrition sweets and snacks.[10] Children's shows rely even more on food advertising since toys are their only other source of revenue, while adult shows attract a wide variety of products. In a mere four hours of Saturday morning cartoons, one study counted over 200 ads for sugared cereals, candy, cookies and chips.[11] That's more than eight commercials for unhealthy foods every ten minutes!

Food ads increase both immediate and long-term consumption of junk food. The sight of food triggers reflexes telling the body, "Now is the time to eat." When our Stone Age ancestors saw freshly cooked meat or a morsel of something sweet in front of them, they ate it then or it was gone. Even two-dimensional images goad appetite. Viewers who see food advertised are likely to get up and grab a bag of something similar—if it's not already at hand next to the remote. People eat more while watching television than during any other leisure activity—mostly low-nutrition sweets and snacks.

Of course the ads do also work in the intended manner: even though the particular food advertised may not be what you grab at that moment, you become likelier to purchase it the next time you're in the store. Even the junk food which is by definition not at hand—takeout burgers, fries and shakes—is consumed more by frequent television viewers. Fresh fruits and vegetables, not much advertised on TV, are consumed in larger quantities by less frequent television viewers.[12]

Maybe you only watch cable or DVDs on your television screen. Perhaps you live in one of the seven million homes equipped with TiVo or another recording device which eliminates ads.[13] Think you're avoiding junk-food shilling? You've only escaped the overt ads. Most readers are at least dimly aware of what the entertainment industry calls "product placement" and what watchdog groups term "covert advertising": brand-name foods, liquor, cigarettes and other products inserted into films and television shows for a fee. However, you may not be aware of its extent.

Old-time Hollywood directors were paid to feature cigarettes in their films. Sometimes a tobacco industry trade conglomerate gave them money simply to see stars smoking. Other times specific manufacturers paid them to place that brand in the hero's hand. Deals in the early days were often a wad of cash and a handshake, so the extent of paid placements will never be fully known. Tobacco companies often denied it. It is now well documented that during the same year in which Phillip Morris claimed it did not engage in product placement, the company inked a half-million-dollar contract with Sylvester Stallone to use their cigarettes in his films.[14]

There were no limits on this until the 1980 film *Superman II* featured a score of intrusive appearances by Marlboro cigarettes: Lois Lane smoked them, their billboards filled aerial fight scenes and a villain locked Superman inside a Marlboro delivery truck. This last detail was especially bizarre, as Marlboro owned no such trucks; tobacco companies feared identification would make them a target for hijackings. The film's prop crew created giant trucks with Marlboro logos. This was deemed so offensive in a "children's" film that it mobilized not only the usual tobacco opponents but also numerous parent groups and spurred restrictions on the placement of tobacco products in films.

There are still no limits on junk food product placements, however, despite an equally lengthy history. The paper trail again tells only part of the story. Film industry archives document that money changed hands for Marilyn Monroe's nibbling Bell potato chips in *The Seven Year Itch* and for multiple appearances of Coca-Cola in 1950's *Father of the Bride*. However, boxes of Sunshine Hi-Hos and Sunshine Grahams prominently lining a shelf above Bette Davis in *All About Eve* are destined to remain simply a suspicious detail.[15]

Product placement is better documented in recent years— and it's taking off. Films got a big green light to be as obtrusive as they liked when *ET* with its Reese's-Pieces-gobbling alien, made a fortune for both film and candy. Spielberg first approached executives at M&Ms, but in one of history's major advertising blunders they declined the deal. Hershey's paid $1 million for the film tie-in and sales of Reese's Pieces soared 80 percent in the following year.[16]

Television was slow to warm up to product placement—until recently. During the 2003–05 seasons, *American Dreams* featured Campbell's Soup, Kraft Singles and Oreos as major parts of the show. One character ghostwrote entries to the Campbell's Soup competition for friends across multiple episodes. On the 2005 season premiere of *Will and Grace*, a character who'd been missing is discovered in hiding, kept alive by another character bringing him not just any sandwiches but an exclusive diet of Subway Chicken Parmigiana sandwiches.[17] Comedy Central's *Shorties Watchin' Shorties* adult cartoon has hosted as paid guests Domino's Pizza and Red Bull energy drink.[18]

Specialty genres have gone further with covert advertising. Reality shows actively solicit paid product placements. On the first episode of the smash hit *Survivor*, the special challenge winners were rewarded with six-packs of Mountain Dew and bags of Doritos. By 2005, *Survivor* teams were receiving Pringles. Many food brands made paid appearances on the NBC reality show *The Restaurant*, about a start-up Manhattan eatery. David Leby, advertising sales director for Turner Broadcasting, brags of *The Real Gilligan's Island*, a reality show based on the 1960s sitcom, that "It lends itself to product placement—funny things wash up on shore."[19] Reality-show product placements can be as simple as the Coca-Cola cups on *American Idol* or as elaborate as NBC's *The Apprentice*, which challenged contestants to design marketing campaigns for Burger King, Domino's Pizza and Nescafe.[20] These were completely integrated into the plot so that discussions about advertisers could occupy enormous blocks of airtime without seeming out of place.

The other genre in which paid placements are ubiquitous is the daytime soap opera. ABC's *All My Children* characters drink Florida orange juice. CBS's *As the World Turns* features Thanksgiving Butterball turkeys. And NBC's *Days of Our Lives* breakfasts on Frosted Flakes.

The 2005 *Advertising Week* panel on product placement was picketed by television writers. Were they protesting the existence of such covert advertising deals? No, they were demanding a cut of the profits. "You can write in anything if you're clever enough," declares Megan McTavish, scriptwriter for *All My Children*. She should know; she recently wrote a passage in which a woman discusses a new Wal-Mart perfume at her comatose husband's bedside—mandatory, as the fragrance's release was set for the date of that episode.[21]

Advertisers already offer payment directly to songwriters, who have more control over their material than television writers. In 2005, McDonald's offered rap singers deals to write Big Macs into their lyrics. Under these contracts, the singers receive no money up front but earn between one and five dollars every each time their song is played on regular or satellite radio.

McDonald's hopes to have a number of these songs playing by the end of 2006. Other advertisers already have rap hits. Seagram's gin received a baldly cynical endorsement in Petey Pablo's "Freek-A-Leek." In one of the most played hip-hop songs of 2004, the rapper proclaims, "Now I got to give a shout-out to Seagram's gin / 'Cause I drink it, and they payin' me for it."

Product placement is effective. A study of the American Music Awards coverage found a 34 percent increase in awareness of brands featured during the show.[22] Viewers exposed to both product placement and traditional advertising during the show were most likely to say they planned to go out and buy the product showcased. Spending on product placement in 2005 totaled $4.25 billion, up from $3.46 billion in 2003.[23]

Networks know that viewers may be hostile to covert advertising. CBS executives have stated that CBS doesn't accept paid placements. This is disingenuous, as the companies producing shows which CBS buys do—CBS airs both *Survivor* and *As the World Turns*. Other comments are more open; Leslie Moonves, chairman of CBS, has predicted in recent months that there will be a "quantum leap in the number of product placements" and that "in one to two years nearly every show on network television will have them."[24]

"Nothing in Moderation"

There's one fast-increasing type of show in which the eating doesn't have to be woven into the plot nor the products "placed." "Nothing in Moderation" is the motto of the International Federation of Competitive Eating (IFOCE). During IFOCE's recently televised Brat-Eating World Championship, Sonya "The Black Widow" downed thirty-five bratwursts in ten minutes—about 10,000 calories. She holds a previous record for consuming eleven pounds of cheesecake in ten minutes.

Established in 1997, the IFOCE has taking the eating contest —an occasional carnival novelty—and turned it into high-grossing television programming. Nathan's Hot Dog Eating Contest, the Wing Bowl and the Krystal Square Off World Hamburger Eating Championship have now been witnessed by millions of "sports" enthusiasts. IFOCE created the Tour de Gorge and over one hundred new competitions for everything from matzo balls to Spam.[25] The athletes have names like "The Locust" and "Cookie" Jarvis. Many are obese—Jarvis weighs between 400 and 500 pounds. Others, including "The Black Widow," are small and train by drinking gallons of water.[26]

And they do call them "athletes." "Without any question, I think of it as a sport," says George Shea, IFOCE chairman. "Eating contests have been around for hundreds of years, and in my belief we are more fundamental and basic and essential than many other sports, such as tennis, which in my opinion is somewhat frivolous."[27]

Indeed, much of the competitive eating programming is on sports channels. Perhaps viewers can no longer bear to witness the levels of physical exertion expended at poker tournaments?

Physicians have their own take on the designation of these events as "sports." "That's preposterous," says gastroenterologist James Smith. "It seems repulsive to call it that." "It certainly doesn't set a good precedent that we are promoting and using as entertainment binge eating," says Joseph P. Regan, a bariatric surgeon.[28]

IFOCE's Shea insists that they sponsor events conducted in a healthy, safe manner. The "athletes" tell a different story. "I'll stretch my stomach until it causes internal bleeding," says "Moses" Lerman, a forty-five-year-old former matzo-ball- and burger-eating champ. "I do it for the thrill of competition. Some people are good at math. Some people are good at golf. I'm good at eating." In typical sports swagger he continues, "When you've eaten your twelfth matzo ball in under three minutes, you have to reach deep within yourself to finish number thirteen."[29]

While food companies are cautious about affixing their product names to something widely considered repulsive, many of the events are paid for by the products being consumed. Who else would sponsor such an event? Well . . . the name of one three-hour yearly special on ESPN is the Alka-Seltzer US Open of Competitive Eating. And, significantly, more than half the IFOCE events are on premium channels, where viewers rather than advertisers foot the bill. Even though it occupies essentially freak-show status now, the number of hours of programming for competitive eating has grown faster over the last three years than for any other type of show.[30]

Heavy Viewers

Television viewing correlates with obesity and weight-related health problems at every age. An article in *Pediatrics* reported that the more television one- to four-year-olds watch, the more likely they are to be overweight.[31] A similar study of five- to eleven-year-olds found the same result and emphasized that effects begin with even one hour of television.[32] The correlation of weight and television viewing continues through adolescence. A study published in the *Journal of the American Medical Association* found that black and Hispanic teens and white girls watch more TV than their white male peers—and they're also heavier. But white males who watched as much television as their minority and female peers were as likely to be obese.

Television correlates with weight-related health problems in childhood, and this becomes even more pronounced for adults. A Harvard study found that men who spent forty hours per week watching television were twice as likely to get diabetes as those who watched under two hours per week.[33] The Nurses' Health Study, a long-term examination of 100,000 women, included data on who became obese and/or diabetic. Each two-hour-per-day

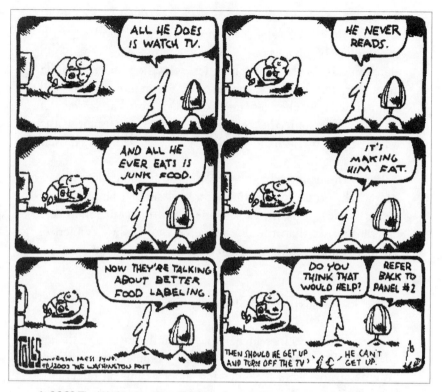

(© 2003 The Washington Post, Toles)

increment in television watching was associated with a 23 percent increase in obesity and a 14 percent increase in diabetes.[34]

Some critics argue that correlations don't prove causation—
and it's plausible that some of the effect is in the other direction, i.e., that as one gets fatter, other activities become more
difficult while television viewing remains easy. The Nurses
study, however, demonstrated that television watching pre-
cedes weight gain. Other studies document that the mechanism for the gain is at least partly the added junk food
consumed in front of the set. Finally, there are a few studies

showing that when you persuade people to cut their television viewing, they lose weight. Stanford educators, working with two groups of elementary school students, gave one group eighteen lessons about watching less television and required a mandatory ten-day-television turn-off. Seven months later, the children who watched less television had gained an average of two pounds less and the average circumference of their waists was nearly an inch smaller than the group who continued their usual viewing habits.[35]

Before discussing other television turn-off studies, let's review a few of the other reasons this might be desirable. There are elements of television content that affect health and fitness in very different senses than the one we've been discussing. Violence, suicidality and reckless driving are health hazards, too.

Sixty Acts of Violins an Hour?

In 1980, Gilda Radner in her role as Emily Lattella, *Saturday Night Live*'s hard-of-hearing political commentator, ranted, "What's all this fuss I keep hearing about violins on television? Why don't parents want their kids to see violins on television? I thought the Leonard Bernstein concerts were just lovely. If they only show violins on television after ten o'clock at night, the little babies will all be asleep and they won't learn any music appreciation. They'll learn to play guitars and bongo drums and join those rock 'n roll outfits. I think there should be *more* violins on television and less game shows. . . ." When Chevy Chase leaned in to whisper that the issue was "violence" on television, Radner muttered her trademark, "Oh well . . . never mind."

The networks apparently never minded either. From the beginning of television, its critics have worried about the effects of violent content on viewers, especially on child viewers. However, at the time of Radner's satire, the most violent prime-time show registered twenty-two acts of violence per hour. More recently, the most violent prime-time show (*Young Indiana Jones*) registered sixty acts of violence per hour.[36]

The average American will witness eight thousand murders and one hundred thousand other acts of violence in a lifetime of television viewing.[37] Eleven thousand of those violent acts will have been seen by the time a child reaches school age. Programs specifically for very young children, such as cartoons, are the most violent of all programming. "Preschoolers have difficulty separating the fantastic from the real," observes child psychiatrist Lillian G. Katz. "Especially when it comes to television fare, its vividness makes even the fantastic seem quite real."[38]

Many studies have found a correlation of real aggression with both television viewing in general and television violence specifically. In a study of the short-term effects, half of a group of children watched an aggressive program; all were then allowed either to facilitate or disrupt another child's game. They could hurt the other child by pressing a button to make the handle which the child was holding hot. The children who had seen the aggressive program were far more aggressive than those who had not.[39] Several studies have confirmed that this holds true for cartoon violence as well as that portrayed by actors.[40]

Zimmerman's study mentioned above in terms of the cognitive effects of television also found that three-year-olds who watch the most television are likeliest to be those that other children identify as bullies at the age of seven.[41] Adolescents' number of hours of television correlate closely with their self-reports of aggressive or antisocial behavior.[42]

Much of the violence in children's shows represents violence as an appropriate way to solve interpersonal problems, to avenge slights and insults, to make up for injustice and to get what you want out of life. A study that highlights the results gave nine- to thirteen-year-old boys and girls situations such as the following: Suppose that you are riding your bicycle down the street and some other child comes up and pushes you off your bicycle. What would you do? The response options included physical or verbal aggression along with options to reduce or avoid conflict. Physical or verbal aggressive responses were selected by 45 percent of heavy-television-violence viewers, compared to only 21 percent of the light-violence viewers.[43]

A study focused on adults examined the effects of suicides in television soap operas on the suicide rate in the United States, using death records compiled by the National Center for Health Statistics. Over a six-year period, each time a major soap-opera personality committed suicide on a television show, within three days there was a significant increase in the number of female suicides across the nation.[44]

Critics of these studies, again, point out that correlation does not prove causation—children who are destined for some biological or environmental reason to be more violent may be drawn to violence on television. However, much as with the Canadian study of the cognitive effects of introducing television, there is a real-life, long-term study looking at the effect of television viewing on violence. After the introduction of television in South Africa in 1974, the murder rate among the white population increased by 56 percent over the next nine years.[45] Though interracial murders—which climbed also—might be attributed to increasing tensions over apartheid, the white-on-white violence has no other easy explanation; most commentators think at least some of it can be blamed on television.

In a study of aggression in children, a San Jose, California, elementary school reduced television viewing by one-third for an entire school year. Parentally installed devices controlled how many hours sets could remain on. By the end of the year, the school had 25 percent fewer fights. A control elementary school that did not reduce the same rate of television viewing experienced no drop in aggression from September to April.[46]

The scientific consensus is clear: "The conclusion of the

public health community, based on over thirty years of research, is that viewing entertainment violence can lead to increases in aggressive attitudes, values and behavior, particularly in children." This is the wording of a 2000 joint position statement to Congress from six professional groups including the American Medical Association and the American Psychological Association.[47]

White Guys Driving Badly

There are many other disturbing aspects of television content. One that is much like violence in terms of its potential for imitation is the high rate of "irregular driving" on television—squealing brakes, speeding, screeching tires and property damage. Physical injuries from such driving and legal penalties are rare, however, especially for likable protagonists.[48]

Most of the groups who are discriminated against in our society are underrepresented on prime-time television. On prime-time television, men outnumber women at least three to one, while in the real world there are slightly more women than men.[49] There are smaller proportions of children, elderly, blacks, Hispanics and other minorities on television than in the real US population.[50] And, of course, there are many fewer overweight or obese people on television than walking around the real world. Frequent, conspicuous scenes of devouring high-calorie foods never result in characters gaining weight.

The list of egregious aspects of television content is too long to detail fully in a book focused primarily on weight and fitness. However, violence, impulsiveness and poor attention impair health and shorten our lifespan, too—and by means that exploit instincts that were adaptive until modern times. All of the content television lures us with has an element of the supernormal stimulus. We're wired to pay close attention to fast movements, emotional outbursts, violence and sexually enticing behavior. Television has hijacked all these potent cues for attention to get us to carefully watch a plastic box with a bunch of wires in it.

What about the *Real* Violins on TV?

By now many readers have probably thought: "But what about the worthwhile shows on television? It's not all violence and car chases. That's not the kind of show I watch!" The categories of shows which people usually argue for as "good" television are 1) the educational—presenting facts or cultural experiences, and 2) the "feel-good" shows about families enjoying life's minor adventures or groups of friends hanging out exchanging amusing banter.

As I've discussed, "educational television" for young children is an oxymoron. Toddlers learn by moving, vocalizing, interacting and getting feedback. From any sort of television, they learn to be passive. Adults can, of course, learn by passively attending to material. But television is a slow way to present content. Yes, you find useful facts about world politics, natural history, home repair and healthy cooking if you select your television shows well—but you could learn in less than five minutes of reading the same content that will occupy a half-hour show. People enjoy getting the information from a charismatic gourmet chef or home repair expert who smiles at the screen and chats in a collegial manner—but that brings us to what's insidious about the "feel-good" shows.

It's not coincidental that the most popular show on US television for years was named *Friends*. *Cheers* used the slogan "Where everybody knows your name." Numerous hits from *I Love Lucy* to *Sex and the City* feature a small group of lively, warm, fun people hanging out, making the viewer feel part of the group. They also spend a remarkable portion of their time eating.

Many scenes in *Friends* are set in the coffee shop where one character waitresses and the rest join her in consuming giant muffins. The *Sex in the City* characters—all pencil thin—regularly rendezvous at their favorite restaurant to devour French fries and desserts while discussing men and Manolo Blahnik shoes.

Parents may like to think that the children's versions of feel-good shows model desirable behavior, but they present pat, unrealistic interactions and solutions—and again, children learn by doing. For adults, these shows target the instinctive drive we have to seek out friendly, supportive people and channel it toward supernormal substitutes for socializing. As White Dot (more about this group in a minute) puts it in a colorful rant:

> What if you turned on *Seinfeld*, only to see Jerry and the gang locked in their separate apartments, watching television. Would that be a good show? Think about it: that's how you are living now. . . . You are alone in the dark, staring at a plastic box. This is like a science fiction horror story. . . . Jerry and Elaine, Kramer, none of them know you. They don't care whether you live or die. Why don't you get yourself some real friends?[51]

Readers of this book probably watch less than the average three hours, more of it may be PBS than network, and you probably do have "real friends." But television still takes you away from them. As we've already discussed in terms of sports in the exercise chapter, watching performances on television competes both with getting out and attending local events—be it Bach or baseball—and with trying activities themselves. People used to walk to concerts or games together and socialize before and after. There wasn't such a huge gap between professionals and audience, so people were likely to meet their favorite players and to try picking up a ball or clarinet themselves. Now local concerts and sports have increasing trouble finding funding, and many seats sit empty at performances.

Two recent studies have found very specific effects of television sets in bedrooms. In one survey of 523 couples in Italy, couples with a television in their bedroom reported having sex half as often as couples without one. Couples under fifty without the bedroom television averaged twice a week, or eight times a month, compared to four times a month for those with a television. For those over fifty, the effect is even more pronounced: seven times a month for those without the television, 1.5 times a month for the television-in-bedroom crowd.[52] A similar study of 2,000 couples in Chicago found that a television in the bedroom correlated most highly with reports of low sexual intimacy, but also correlated with lower conversational and emotional intimacy.[53]

Turn It Off

After researching the ill effects of television on mood, creativity, concentration and fitness, Robert Kubey and Mihaly Csikszentmihalyi conclude, "That does not mean that watching television, per se, is problematic . . . the difficulty arises when people strongly sense that they ought not to watch as much as they do and yet find themselves strangely unable to reduce their viewing."

I disagree. The findings of Kubey, Csikszentmihalyi and other researchers *do* imply that television per se is problematic. More is worse, but the negative effect on health is there at any level. Gallup polls during both 1992 and 1999 found that two out of five adults and seven out of ten teenagers thought they spent too much time watching television. Ten percent of adults consider themselves TV addicts. But many more are watching four to ten hours a day and getting no exercise without "strongly sensing they ought not to watch as much." Just as with food, humans can't always simply listen to their instincts in the face of modern supernormal stimuli. Media scholars, like diet experts, shy away from prescribing something "too extreme" that "no one will follow." Common advice is to cut viewing by an hour a day and stick to your favorite shows. However, as with junk food and other addictions, it is often harder to cut back a little than to quit. Numerous studies document that when someone turns on a television set "for this one show," it often stays on for hours.

There have been several "cold-turkey" television withdrawal experiments. Some paid families to turn off their televisions for periods of a month or more. Others followed participants in the annual "turn off your television" week that we'll discuss more in the next section. These studies find remarkably good outcomes as people have adjustment problems *very briefly*. As one review of these studies summarized:

> The first three or four days for most persons were the worst, even in many homes where viewing was minimal and where there were other ongoing activities. In over half of all the households, during these first few days of loss, the regular routines were disrupted, family members had difficulties in dealing with the newly available time, anxiety and aggressions were expressed . . . People living alone tended to be bored and irritated.

Family logs from the first few days of one study included the following entries: "The family walked around like a chicken without a head"; "Children bothered me, and my nerves were on edge. Tried to interest them in games, but impossible. TV is part of them"; and, more ironically, "It was terrible. We did nothing— my husband and I talked." Most of the dropouts, even in the long-term studies, were within these first three days.

Very soon—within days—the former television viewers adapt and rediscover their enjoyment of many other activities. Families begin to play games, take walks and talk more.

Television Turn-Off

Television Turn-Off Week began in 1994. This early April event is promoted in over a dozen countries by groups including the US TV Turnoff Network, Britain's White Dot (named for the lingering image just after the set has been turned off) and Canada's Adbusters. Some cities have local promotions, such as NY Unplugged. These groups distribute pamphlets through schools and libraries encouraging families to participate. They offer events such as picnics and bike rides and lists of do-on-your-own activities. Both the past two US Surgeons General—C. Everett Koop and David Satcher—have endorsed TV Turn-Off Week.

Young adult events for the week have ranged from a "Smash Your Set" punk concert in Vancouver to a street drama "TV zombie invasion" in New York City. Many of the television turn-off groups have guerrilla branches that organize outings to restaurants, bars and malls to turn off public sets. These utilize the TV-B-Gone, a 1½-inch universal television remote which turns off virtually any television within a range of 20 to 50 feet. Some public turn-off groups use the tiny device surreptitiously; others zap sets blatantly while handing out turn-off literature.

"People may think it is intrusive for an anti-television campaigner to go into a [bar] and turn off the television, but a lot of people find the television intrusive," observes the inventor of the device, Mitch Altman, a forty-eight-year-old former TV addict who hasn't owned a television since 1980. The TV-B-Gone website promotes it for the individual anti-television crusader also: "Safe. Fun. Effective. . . . Imagine sports bars or

annoying talking head shows that appear on monitors at the airport. Add to that your own creativity and we're pretty sure
you'll come up with some ideas."[54] The website points out that
the TV-B-Gone is blocked by solid walls but can pass through
window glass, so it's probably been applied in maneuvers a bit
more intrusive than silencing public sets. With an advertising
budget of zero, Altman has sold 40,000 of the devices.

In 2004, an estimated 7.6 million children and adults partic-
ipated in over 19,000 organized turn-offs in every state in the
US. Generally the response is positive—and remember, the
research suggests that the difficult withdrawal period would
occupy half the week. Some reviews are mixed: "I really didn't
like TV Turn-Off Week except that I did notice that my grades
went up and I was in a good mood all week," comments one
second-grader from Donora, Pennsylvania.[55]

Cold Turkey

Dropping television is an ideal companion to a new diet and
exercise regime. If you insist that television needs to be part of
your healthy lifestyle, I suggest you place a stationary bike or
treadmill in front of it and attach one of those devices that turns
off the set if your pace lags. We've all seen television sets in
front of exercise machines that just get sat on or peered over
from the couch—you really need the set to turn off when you're
not in motion. I don't mean that rare one-in-a-hundred person
who watches only one show a week or who already pedals vig-
orously through one hour a day of viewing. As with the one-
chocolate-a-month anomaly, I wouldn't argue with success. I
mean the ninety-nine in a hundred.

TV Turn-Off advocates that people turn off their sets for one
week. I recommend doing so permanently. An hour a day
toward physical activity, an hour a week toward shopping at

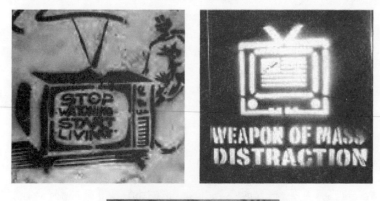

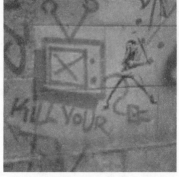

Stenciled graffiti appears on a wall in Glasgow, Scotland; a phone booth in Santa Fe, New Mexico; a basement club in Barcelona; and various walls across the United States. *(Top left: photo by Brian Aslak Gylte. Top right: photo by Ron Kaufman. Both courtesy of www.turnoffyourtv.com. Bottom: photo by Sean Cartoon)*

that little farmers' market—and the remainder for any creative, social or professional pursuit you somehow haven't been finding time for.

That study about whether four- and five-year-old children would rather give up their father or their television? Many people are surprised that dads are actually winning, almost two to one.[56] Nevertheless, we can do better; let's widen that gap.

6

You Can't Be Too Rich
or Too Thin

Subject: Beautiful Women

From: *AnyWoman@server.com*

To: *AnyOtherWoman@server.com*

06/01/Every year

Did you know that it's Beautiful Women Month? Well it is and that means you and me.

I'm supposed to send this to FIVE BEAUTIFUL WOMEN, and you are one of them!!!

Did you know that in 1921, Miss America had a body mass index of 20.4? By 1986, it was 16.8.

That Marilyn Monroe wore a size 14? [size 16 in some versions of the email]

That if shop mannequins were real women they'd be too thin to menstruate?

That 20 years ago, models weighed 8% less than the average woman? Today they weigh 23% less.

That the Venus of Willendorf statue of a goddess from the Stone Age would be classified as morbidly obese by today's standards?

Have you received this email? For the past seven years, it has been forwarded to hundreds of thousands of women—and the occasional man. The fascination with these "facts" lies in their implication that our current equation of beauty with slimness is so extreme and so uniquely modern that great beauties of earlier eras would be dismissed as "fat" today. The implicit message is that it is dangerous and futile to strive for today's ideal—and that senders and readers of the email might have been considered great beauties but for the cruel timing of their birth.

Susie Orbach's *Fat Is a Feminist Issue*[1] and the literature of the National Association to Advance Fat Acceptance (NAAFA) express similar beliefs about the arbitrary and misguided nature of society's ideal for weight. It's easy to sympathize with the politics behind such messages, but are they true? Sympathy is no reason to accept bad arguments—arguments that ignore history, medical research and basic evolutionary principles.

There is indeed much to decry about the effects of beauty pageants and modern media on women's self-image. However, promoting unhealthy thinness—or even much more thinness than was preferred in past eras—isn't among their offenses. I'm going to address the email "facts" as examples of what's wrong with this whole line of argument. I'll show that today's ideal and those of past eras are about the same. The email—and indeed many implications of physical attractiveness—are specific to women, but I'll discuss the extent to which they apply or differ for men. Finally, I'll challenge the idea that standards of beauty are arbitrary or could derail us from the pursuit of health. I'll argue that they reflect our evolutionary need to estimate the health of others from their physical characteristics. Humans would have died off long ago if the ideal female body couldn't menstruate.

Beautiful Women Email "Fact" Check

Miss America's BMI. The statement citing a higher body mass index* in 1920 versus a lower one in 1986 could as easily have read, "Miss America had a BMI of 18.9 in 1927, but by 2001 that figure had *risen* to 20.3." All four specific numbers are accurate, but it's trends that matter. The pageant's winners have decreased in weight only very slightly from its inception to the present.[2] More specifically, they dropped a bit from 1920 through 1980, then regained most of that small difference. Except for the first and last decades, with fewer contestants and a less reliable average (the 1920s with an average BMI of 21 and the 2000s with an average BMI of 20), all other decades fall within the narrow range of 18.25–19.5. Even these small differences diminish when one controls for height and age: Miss America has been getting taller and older over time. That 1921 winner whose BMI is cited in the email was also 5'1" and sixteen years old! The main BMI guidelines explicitly state that they're not relevant for anyone under eighteen; there are separate, *lower* ones for adolescents.

More unvarying yet than BMI, Miss America's waist-to-hip ratio has always hugged .7. This proportion has been cited as an unvarying body ideal in art through the centuries.[3] As I'll discuss in the next chapter on health, waist-to-hip ratio may be an even better predictor of both aesthetics and health than BMI, though it correlates strongly with that index. It's much easier to have a low waist-to-hip ratio at a lower weight. Because of this correlation and because the Miss America pageant is one of only a few settings where exact measurements are known, I'll continue to discuss weight mainly in terms of BMI through this chapter.

*Body mass index is discussed in detail in Chapter 7.

Miss Monroe's dress size. From the 1950s to today, the measurements designating a particular size have grown as the weight of the average woman has increased. This is most obvious with "small," "medium" and "large": most women don't want to wear a "large"; therefore, "medium" is assigned to whatever size the average woman fits into. This size drift has happened with the numbered system also. Women who've gained thirty pounds during their adult lives can be heard to say, "I still wear the same dress size I did when I was eighteen." They're likely to be telling the truth. A 1950s size 14 has the dimensions of today's 10; a 1950s 16 is today's 12.

Most people's weight fluctuates, and Marilyn was no exception. Early in her career, her press releases claimed she weighed 118 pounds, which looks plausible for the slender girl in *Ladies of the Chorus*. By her last two films, her publicist wasn't advertising Marilyn's weight, but measurements on her gowns from that era would suggest it may have climbed as high as 140.

On the rare occasions when Marilyn bought ready-made clothes, she probably purchased 1950s size 14 or 16—today's size 10–12. But ready-mades were invariably altered to hug her hourglass figure. On average, Marilyn was wearing the equivalent of the bust of a modern size 12, the hips of an 8 and the waist of a 4.

Philippe Halsman's 1952 candid photo of Marilyn is equally discouraging of the other myth that beauties of past eras didn't work at maintaining their figures. Weight training may have been the exception, but most swam laps or played tennis. Many actresses were competent tap or chorus-line dancers. Marilyn wrestled with depression and addiction, downing barbiturates with booze and remaining in bed all day intermittently throughout her mid- to late career. However, through much of her life she was active and fit.

Mannequins "too thin to menstruate." A brief review of mannequins listed for sale on the Internet[4] yields a narrow range

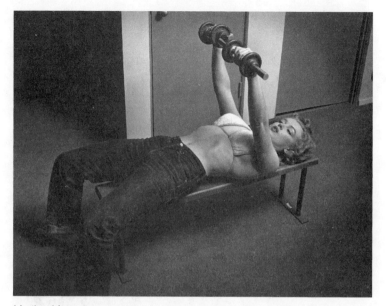

Marilyn Monroe:
   Height, 5' 5½"
   Weight, 118–140 pounds
   Bust, 35"–37"
   Waist, 22"–23"
   Hips, 36"–37"
(Photo by Philippe Halsman © Halsman Estate)

of heights and measurements (weight being obviously irrelevant for fiberglass women). New mannequins are similar to Miss America's proportions—waist sizes almost exactly the same and chest and hips about an inch smaller than the real women. Those listed by dress size were all described as either "size 6" or "size 4–6." If they were flesh-and-blood women, they'd have an approximate BMI of 18.3. Just as with Miss America, when one compares mannequins from an earlier era, there's a modern trend toward taller bodies rather than lighter ones—but it's a small difference.

Fertility sites warn that women with a BMI of less than 17

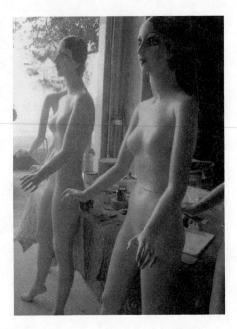

Mannequins from the 1920s have much the same dimensions as those of today. *(Photo by Shelly Freeman, The Mannequin Gallery)*

may have more difficulty conceiving than those of average weight. None of the mannequins fall in this range, and a BMI below 17 is hardly a total rule-out for menstruation or fertility anyway. High-BMI women have greater problems conceiving.

"Twenty years ago, models weighed 8 percent less than the average woman. Today they weigh 23 percent less." Which group do you think has significantly changed during that time?

Fashion models have always had BMIs around 17–18, slightly thinner than the averages for Miss America or for actresses. A few models indeed have eating disorders or keep their weight down with drugs. These burn out their careers by thirty or even die by that age like HIV-positive, heroin-addicted supermodel Gia Carangi, who inspired the biopic *Gia* in which she was portrayed by Angelina Jolie. However, the vast majority of models maintain their weight with a low-calorie diet and lots of exer-

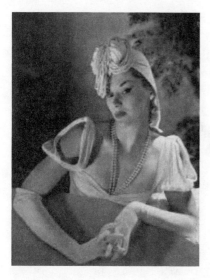

Lisa Fonssagrives-Penn (1911–92) has been dubbed "the first super-model." Her image graced the covers of *Vogue, Vanity Fair* and *Town and Country* in the 1930s, 1940s and 1950s. In a *Life* interview, she gave tips on how she maintained her seventeen-inch waist: Ms. Fonssagrives-Penn ate numerous but very small meals— six grapes, one cracker, one slice of cheese and a swallow of wine being typical. *(Photo by Ferdinand Fonssagrives)*

cise, and they enjoy excellent health. Twiggy—who was fre-quently criticized in the 1960s as the epitome of supposedly "unhealthy thin"—is still modeling today, as are Christie Brink-ley, now in her fifties, and Lauren Hutton, in her sixties. These women are healthy, energetic—and still slim.[5]

The Venus of Willendorf. This is a much more intriguing representation of the female body than those store mannequins. One can't calculate the BMI of a three-inch limestone carving exactly, but it's fair to estimate that her flesh-and-blood equiv-alent would fall in the morbidly obese range. But what of the email's statement that she was "a goddess worshipped in the Stone Age"? What do we know about the purpose of this pre-historic carving? The short answer is nothing.

Paleolithic carved women were first referred to as "Venuses" jokingly, when the Venus of Laugerie Basse was discovered in 1864. The term "Venus pudica" or "modest Venus" referred to a type of Roman statue in which the goddess is attempting to conceal her breasts and pubic area from view. Because the Laugerie Basse figure had detailed genitalia that she made no attempt to hide, its discoverer playfully reversed the term to "Venus impudica" or "immodest Venus." By the time the Willendorf was discovered in 1908, the term had stuck and all Paleolithic carvings were referred to as "Venus figurines."[6]

The Willendorf was dated around 20,000–24,000 BC—the earliest known representation of a human body. It has indeed been discussed by anthropologists as possibly a goddess figure.

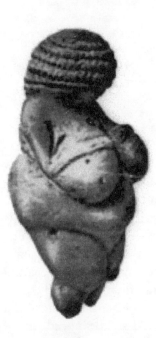

Some "experts" declare that it is definitely a religious artifact, others that it is clearly not of a non-religious nature.[7] Some see the figure as obviously pregnant; others claim, with equal certainty, that the amount of fat over her hips compared with her stomach suggests a very heavy non-pregnant young woman. No one thinks her figure could have been average for the Stone Age—skeletal evidence makes clear otherwise. Opinions vary, however, as to whether she's intended as a realistic representation of an unusual body or a stylized version of a more typical one.

Some anthropologists believe the figure may indeed have been an ideal. They speculate that when food was scarcer corpulence may have been desirable as an indicator of status. Others view it as a possible caricature—like the

Venus of Willendorf. *(Venus of Willendorf, 24,000–22,000 BCE, Oolitic limestone 11.1 cm, courtesy of Naturhistorisches Museum, Vienna)*

modern kewpie doll. Noting that it easily fits into one hand, some suggest that she might have been a masturbatory object for men—the Stone Age equivalent of *Playboy*. Yet others invoke the same hand-sized quality as implying she might have been a child's doll. One speculates that she may have been intended to be "inserted into the vagina, perhaps as a fertility ritual."[8] The more one reads of the commentary about the lady of Willendorf, the more she resembles the Rorschach ink blots—telling us more about the beholder than about the artisan or model of twenty-five thousand years ago.

The email and other popular discussions of the Venus of Willendorf ignore two characteristics that are as striking as her weight. First, she has no face—which makes her an unlikely embodiment of the feminist ideal. Her head is covered with a spiral of round bumps, alternately interpreted as plaited hair, a caplike cloth covering the face or a representation of some abstract concept we can't fathom.

The second unusual characteristic is that the otherwise obese figure—with her huge rolls of fat across stomach, hips and thighs—has scrawny, emaciated arms. One does not see the equivalent enthusiastic statements about Stone Age people worshipping an ineffectual "goddess" incapable of grasping a five-pound object, or speculation on what form of muscular atrophy was viewed as ideal. Instead, most explanations see the thin arms as a stylization or reflect on the difficulty of using crude tools to carve realistic arms into crumble-prone limestone.

Indeed, the most plausible explanations for her overall weight are the same two that would account for these other characteristics: that she's a stylization meant to emphasize the enlarged areas—breasts, stomach and genitals—and/or that the generally round shape is easiest to carve without breaking the porous stone.[9]

Other Stone Age figures exist. Some are heavy, but not all. As

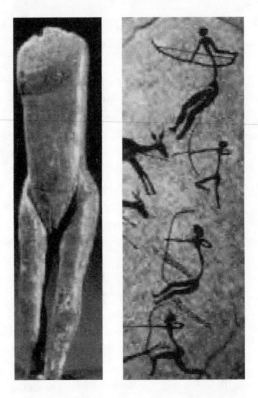

Venus of Laugerie Basse
(left), Lascaux Cave
figures (right). *(Venus
of Laugerie Basse, c.
30,000–26,000 BCE,
Mammoth ivory, 8 cm,
courtesy of Musée de
l'Homme, Paris. Lascaux
Cave Figures, Lascaux
Caves, Lascaux, France)*

we've mentioned, the first one found—seventy-five years before
the Willendorf—and the one originally termed a "Venus figure" is
the Venus of Laugerie Basse. This "Venus" is flat-chested and thin.
Figures in cave paintings from a similar era and region are usually
sticklike. If interpreted literally, they're depicting extremely gaunt
humans.

But again, most experts think the gauntness is at least partly
a function of what's easier to represent with a drawing tool, and
that perhaps the figures are stylized for other reasons.

One Paleolithic "Venus" has a lion's head, and some of the cave
drawings depict people with antlers or other surreal characteristics.
These are clearly neither literal representations nor human ideals.

The Appeal of the Myth

While we can never know exactly what the Venus of Willendorf represented in her own time, it's clearer what she means in ours. The mild version of the Willendorf's message is that many body types are attractive to one's fellow humans. This serves as an antidote to the poor body image many women have, though it's not helpful to imply this was true only in times past; it's true today too. The extreme version of the Willendorf message is more problematic: that a BMI over 30 is a natural ideal which—despite its high cholesterol and diabetic blood sugar—would still be lauded as such today except for some cruel twist of fate—or crueler plot by the media. If you are overweight, it's comforting to think that your figure would have been ideal in another era. The truth is that you might indeed have been closer to the ideal—but only because *you would have been thinner if you had lived in that era*, not because the ideal was heavier.

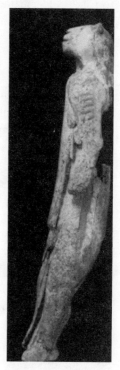

Venus of Hohlenstein-Stadel. *(Venus of Hohlenstein-Stadel, c. 30,000–26,000 BCE, Mammoth ivory, 11¼", courtesy of Ulmer Museum, Ulm, Germany)*

Consider the quote, "Fat is now regarded as an indiscretion, and almost as a crime." A modern magazine examining our values in the new millennium? No, this is from an issue of *Living Age* printed in 1914. Reading *Gone with the Wind*'s description of Scarlett squeezing her corset waist down to the requisite eighteen inches underlines that the ideal wasn't heavier either in the

1860s, when the book is set, or in the 1920s, when it was written. In 1929 Lucky Strike cigarettes decided to target women. Their new ads proclaimed, "Instead of eating between meals . . . instead of fattening sweets . . . beautiful women keep youthful slenderness these days by smoking *Luckies*. . . . For years this has been no secret to those men who keep fit and trim." According to the US Department of Health's tobacco division, "The positioning of Lucky Strikes as a weight-control aid led to a greater than 300% increase of sales for this brand in the first year of the campaign."[10]

In 1924, the *Journal of the American Medical Association* published an article which stated, "Overweight is a mar to beauty. . . . An excess of fat destroys grace and delicacy. . . . A fat face has a monstrous uniformity. No theatrical producer would hire a plump actress to mirror the real depths of the human soul."[11] Can you imagine JAMA printing this today?

This chapter's title, "You Can't Be Too Rich or Too Thin," has been attributed to a number of thin, wealthy women—none of our era: Rose Kennedy, Diana Vreeland, the Duchess of Windsor and Babe Paley. They all seem to have repeated it, and the Duchess had it embroidered on a pillow. However, it originated with a person to whom it's rarely attributed: Truman Capote. Quote maven Alec Lewis says Capote first uttered the phrase on *The David Susskind Show* over fifty years ago.[12]

There is an oft-repeated stereotype that black or Hispanic Americans favor a much heavier ideal than do whites. This does not appear to be true. One study found that blacks on average preferred a female form that was ten pounds heavier than that favored by whites.[13] Three other surveys which polled people of different races about their preferences found that minority women would like to weigh about the same as would white women and that minority men favor the same female body shape as do white men.[14]

A *very* few societies have indeed idealized heavy bodies. In Nigeria, pubertal girls used to be shut in a special "fattening hut" in preparation for marriage.[15] During months of forced inactivity, they consumed large quantities of rice, yams, plantains and porridge. This practice has decreased but remains in some of the same regions of Nigeria that still practice genital excision on girls.[16] The Massa tribe of northern Cameroon historically encouraged young men to gain weight to enhance their appearance.[17] In parts of Polynesia, royalty or other elite of both genders were fattened almost to the point of immobility as a sign of status. During epidemics which emaciate the victims— such as in parts of late eighteenth-century Europe during tuberculosis outbreaks and in AIDS-ravaged African nations today—preference for plumper bodies that are less likely to be harboring the illness is explicitly taught.

More important than these few exceptions where the ideal is heavy is the fact that a wide array of weights have always been seen as appealing—at least as long as other indicators of health are present. The "it's a modern fad" group overemphasizes positive heavy images from the past—pointing out the erotic nudes of Rubens while ignoring those of Modigliani. And they also ignore the range of weights considered attractive in ours. Does anyone think Renée Zellweger at her *Bridget Jones* weight isn't seen as sexy and adorable? Or that the late Anna Nicole Smith wasn't a major object of lust in her plumpish *Playboy* centerfold and Guess jeans model days—and at least an occasional object of lust during the downright obese period of her reality TV show?

The women commonly cited as exceptions to needing to look great in order to get ahead in show business—Oprah Winfrey in her pre-diet days, Rosie O'Donnell, Roseanne Barr—are usually in the next breath contradictorily described as "beautiful." One doesn't need to be ideal in every trait to be

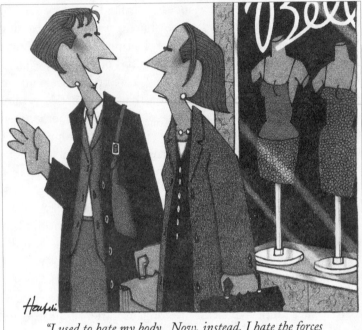

"I used to hate my body. Now, instead, I hate the forces
that conspire to make me hate my body."

(© The New Yorker Collection 2000 William Haefeli from cartoonbank.com)

viewed as marvelously attractive. These women are way ahead
on most aesthetics: smooth, unblemished skin, narrow waists,
wide eyes, small noses, light jaws and radiant smiles.[18] Nor
does one even need to look like these plumper "almost-ideal"
woman to be attractive. Fortunately, quite average-looking
people are visually appealing to their fellow humans. So it's
not meaningful to compare what was seen as potentially
attractive in past eras (most of which still would be) with
modern ideals. The ideals have always been narrower—
including narrower body dimensions.

There are two real changes from past eras. The first relates to the fact that while the ideal remains similar across time, the ease of achieving its components varies. In past eras, when food supplies consisted of smaller quantities and healthy unrefined foods, most people were trim. Smallpox and lesser skin infections were rampant and many people were covered with sores or pock mark scarring. In those times, "smooth" or "unblemished" skin "like a newborn babe's" was often included in descriptions of beauty, and "slender" was less common. Teeth may be a bit of a plus now if they're exceptionally straight and white, but the declaration that "I have all my own teeth," which in past times was a serious asset for a mate, is currently used mostly in jest. Weight is indeed emphasized more now as it represents a more common departure from the ideal.

The second change concerns our tendency to compare ourselves to others. Humans have always evaluated their personal attributes against those of their neighbors, and for women physical appearance was always a large part of these comparisons. What is different now is that the pool of people for potential comparison has grown phenomenally—and only the most unusually attractive are conveyed by the media around the world. Stone Age girls probably wished to be prettier than their few tribal peers, but if you weren't the prettiest girl in the village, the difference wasn't likely to be dramatic. Now society culls from literally millions of young women to select faces and bodies, then perfects these with Adobe Photoshop. The difference between the resulting magazine cover and our average modern girl is staggering.

The goal of the "Beautiful Women" email is laudable—to make women feel better about themselves, to break the hold of this one-in-a-million comparison to which they're subjecting themselves. But it's also misguided. Of course women shouldn't base their self-esteem predominantly on their looks, be they thin or heavy. However, the tendency to compare oneself to others is ancient and the current tendency to emphasize weight is because that's become such a common problem. Denial doesn't help anything—and claiming the average woman's weight is healthy and that models are too thin doesn't make it so.

And, as we've already emphasized, one doesn't have to be anywhere near an ideal weight or ideal anything else to be attractive. But that's not to say that all weights are equal for health purposes and that there's no value in striving to approach the ideal. As one blogger puts it, "Just like I looked up to my women professors in college as intellectual models, I look at fashion models as body models."[19] Presently, there's a widespread indignation at images of beauty that most of us are unable to match, yet we're comfortable with geniuses,

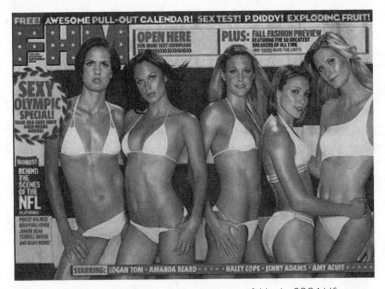

Some of the thinnest women ever to appear as centerfolds: the 2004 US Olympic team. (© *George Holz*)

saints and entrepreneurs whose example may inspire many who won't actually achieve that level of intellect, morality or wealth.

And for those who'd prefer a different sort of "body model," the women who finish marathons or win basketball championships are similarly lean. Women athletes indeed averaged a bit heavier in past decades— but they also averaged a bit slower.

Men's appearance has never played as great a role

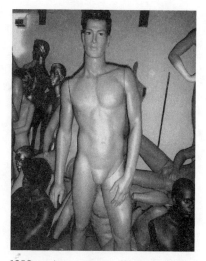

1950s male mannequin. *(Photo by Shelly Freeman, The Mannequin Gallery)*

as women's in their status or desirability as a mate. However, there is nevertheless a common myth that, to the extent there is a preferred body type for men, it has changed recently. One variation on this claim is that the male ideal is "recently" slim—that, as with women, it used to be plumper. The other variation claims there is an equivalent "new" emphasis on muscle definition and tone, while the male ideal used to be less muscular. Indeed, then and now, more male actors vary from any physical ideal more than do their female counterparts simply because physical attractiveness isn't weighted as heavily for men as charisma, status and achievements. But when we look at the pure version of the physical ideal—those plaster or plastic store mannequins—they tell a different story. The ideal was always just as muscular and just as thin, though not as thin as for women: the male mannequin generally translates to a BMI of 20 or 21.

So our preference for thinness isn't new—it has been there across centuries and cultures. Why is this? In the next chapter we'll examine the medical data on BMI which begins to answer this question. Our aesthetic ideals are—as evolutionary theory would predict they must be—essentially "the picture of health."

7

The Bearable Lightness of Being: Medical Views on Ideal Weight

It is often claimed that modern society is "obsessed" with weight and dieting, but this is true only to the extent that many more of us are in a weight range that would have been a concern in most eras. Medical articles tout "new discoveries" of the relationship between excess weight and a variety of illnesses. This is like tobacco companies saying that the risks of smoking were unearthed only by recent research despite generations of people referring to cigarettes as "coffin nails" and chronic lung congestion as "smokers' cough."

Common sense and simple observation have long noted a relationship between excess weight and health problems. In 400 BC Hippocrates wrote, "Persons who are constitutionally very fat are apt to die earlier than those who are slender."[1] His Roman counterpart, Celsus, agreed: "Many of the obese are throttled by acute disease and difficulty breathing; they die often suddenly which rarely happens in a thinner person."[2] A century ago, one popular medical book observed simply, "A fat man is an unhealthy man,"[3] while another elaborated, "He may suffer from fatty diabetes, gouty hypertension, from hepatitis or enteritis, from cardiac, varicose or renal troubles, but he will always be an old man before his time."[4] "To Lengthen thy Life, Lessen thy Meals," advised Benjamin Franklin in *Poor Richard's Almanac*.[5]

Medical weight-loss regimens existed in classical Greece and medieval Europe.[6] In the first-century Greek tome *On the Fat and Lean Mode of Life*, Galen recommended "quick exercise"— he especially favored archery. In one of the earliest applications of behavioral principles, he allowed small amounts of food "to be consumed only after exercise."[7] Paulus of Aegina also advised exercise and small meals—the later "preferably taken only once a day."[8] By the thirteenth century, a text at the medical school of Salerno recommended a similarly restricted diet and increased exercise but also remarked in passing that "vinegar is of no use for obesity,"[9] indicating that that modern bit of alternative-health advice was already circulating. Even for those not overweight, the twelfth-century Jewish physician Maimonides recommended, "One should not eat until one's stomach is full, but one should eat until one's stomach is three-quarters full."[10]

Diet books for the general public have been popular since the invention of the printing press. Probably most famous was William Banting's *Letter on Corpulence*, published in London in the 1840s. It forbade bread, butter, milk, sugar, beer and potatoes—"the most insidious enemies a man, with a tendency to corpulence in advanced life, can possess."[11] *Letter* was a best-seller in Europe for several decades and "banting" became the colloquial term for dieting. Other publications of that period include *Comments on Corpulency*, *The Cure of Obesity* and *Why Be Fat?*[12]

These were European books, and in 1860 physician S. Weir Mitchell observed, "Banting with us Americans is a rarely needed process, as a rule."[13] Within a couple of decades, however, America had caught up to Europe's rich diet and sedentary ways. On both sides of the Atlantic, books appeared which contained most of the components of modern diet advice. Those by Banting and James Salisbury[14] were what we now call "low-carbohydrate." Those by Sylvester Graham and John Kellogg were low-fat, high-carbohydrate, and Lulu Hunt's contained calorie tables much like those found in today's books. Spas with mineral baths that were supposed to "cleanse the body of fat" sprang up, as did health retreats for diet—including one run by Kellogg. These nineteenth- and early twentieth-century authors' names persist in today's foods: graham crackers, Kellogg's cornflakes, and Salisbury steak. The Swedish term for dieting is still "banting."

The Deadliest Sin? Religious Views on Gluttony and Sloth

Another tradition that historically held authority parallel to the medical establishment's is religion. The Christian Bible rebukes those with "slothful bellies"[15] or "whose God is their belly."[16] The sixth-century Pope Gregory the Great placed gluttony on his list of the seven deadly sins—those which consign one's soul to hell. Though all were deadly, Pope Gregory took care to rank them from most serious to least: pride, envy, anger, sloth, greed, gluttony and lust.[17] He censored sins of aggression more harshly than those indulging pleasures—and it's notable that the sins of gluttony and sloth were more serious than lust. For centuries, Christian tradition retained these priorities: in Dante's *Inferno*, the gluttonous are consigned to a lower circle of hell than the lecherous. John Sinclair, who translated Dante into English, explains that this is because gluttony is purely an impulse of the flesh while lust can involve more human and spiritual components.[18]

From a secular and evolutionary viewpoint, the "seven sins"

might be viewed as a list of instincts that were once adaptive but have become "deadly" in our modern settings. For instance, lust would have been appropriate when one encountered only the occasional member of the opposite sex out on the savannah, but it's confusing now that hundreds of alluring bodies can parade past you in one city block. Anger made sense when men had only fists to defend hunting territory, but it doesn't when they have guns and are competing for parking spaces. Pope Gregory's most censored sins are the ones that are most destructive to others, but gluttony is the deadliest for the "sinner."

The *Catholic Encyclopedia* entry for "gluttony" is consistent with this concept of sin as the favoring of instinct over civilized necessity:

> From Lat. *gluttire*, to swallow, to gulp down: the excessive indulgence in food and drink. The moral deformity discernible in this vice lies in its defiance of the order postulated by reason, which prescribes necessity as the measure of indulgence in eating and drinking. . . . Clearly one who uses food or drink in such a way as to injure his health . . . is guilty of the sin of gluttony. . . . It is incontrovertible that to eat or drink for the mere pleasure of the experience . . . is likewise to commit the sin of gluttony.

Sloth, another of Gregory's seven deadly sins, is defined equally literally: "In general it means disinclination to labour or exertion. . . ."

Most religions have periods during which one is supposed to practice special restraint in eating. The Muslim holy month of Ramadan is observed by fasting during daylight hours. Devout Hindus abstain from all food for a day and a half every fortnight as a means of spiritual improvement; the political fasts of Gandhi were inspired by this practice. Jews fast on Yom Kippur

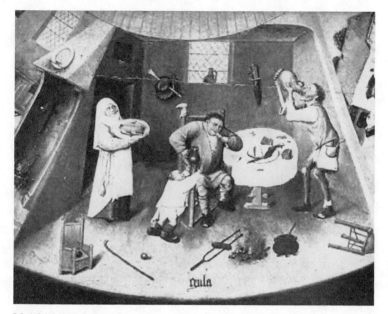

"Gula" (gluttony) detail from Hieronymous Bosch's *Seven Deadly Sins*.

as atonement for sins and on Tishah-b'Ab in memory of tragedies that befell the Jewish people.[19] Lent was a period of food restriction for early Christians. Though there were religious feasts in most of these same traditions, even then there were injunctions against "continuing long at feasts"[20] or being "insatiable" at banquets.[21] Physical labor is required in both Christian and Buddhist monastic orders as a sign of devotion.

In 1522, Protestant reformers rejected Lentian fasting. In the "Affair of the Sausages," several Austrian priests were discovered eating sausage on Ash Wednesday. Instead of meting out severe punishment, the Master of Grossmunster Cathedral in Zurich took the opportunity to decree that Christians should have free choice in the matter of whether to fast. Some

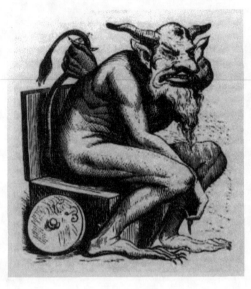

ßelphegor: the demon who often represented sloth incarnate. This sin was at other times represented by scenes of falling asleep on the job, especially if the job was being performed by a monk. *(Eighteenth-century engraving, unknown artist)*

Protestant denominations began to actively condemn fasting as papist. Meanwhile, in 1962 with Vatican II, Catholicism softened its demands for Lentian fasting to simply the elimination of rich foods or the consumption of small meals during this period. Gluttony and sloth are much less discussed in today's churches, though they remain officially sins in the theology of most.

Some modern writings reinterpret sloth as inertia in the spiritual rather than the physical realm—though that was definitely not Pope Gregory's intent. Gregory's description of the characteristics of gluttony sound like routine modern dietary habits:

"sometimes it seeks costly meats; sometimes it requires that food be daintily cooked; sometimes it exceeds the measure of refreshment by taking too much; sometimes we sin by the very heat of an immediate appetite."[22] There is a trend to view gluttony as some exotic behavior achieved only at Roman feasts. "I know gluttony is a bad thing," said the Reverend Jerry Falwell, a heavy man who has been hospitalized for cardiac problems. "But I don't know many gluttons."[23] So much for not eating "more than necessity prescribes" or not using food "in a manner that would harm the body."

Like other societal norms, religious guidelines on diet and exercise have slackened to accommodate followers' lifestyles. The typical fried chicken and cheese casserole church pot-luck is testimony to the no-longer-very-moderating effects of the church on eating. In fact, a 1998 Purdue University study actually found that obesity levels *rose* with higher levels of religious participation.[24] They also found differences among denominations, with Baptists the heaviest, other Protestants next and Catholics in the middle. Jews, Hindus and other non-Christians had the lowest rates of obesity—except, that is, for the lighter yet non-religious. Unlike the strong correlation with religious participation, however, these denominational differences disappeared when researchers controlled for region of the country— more Protestants live in the South and Midwest, which are the heaviest states, while more Catholics and non-Christians live in the Northeast and West Coast, where there is less obesity. It's not clear in this case whether controlling for region of the country makes statistical sense. It would if geography somehow caused weight, but since the denominational differences correspond to the degree to which they emphasize fasting or restraint, religious persuasion may be the more relevant variable. There are a few radical denominations not included in the Purdue study, such as the Amish and Seventh-day Adventists, who still enforce dietary restraint and/or vigorous exercise;

other research has found that their weights are the only ones which stay well below American averages.[25]

The History of Recommended Height and Weight

Medicine has long been interested in an objective definition of "overweight." In 1871, French surgeon Paul Broca published a formula for calculating the ideal weight-by-height for each gender. Translated into pounds and inches for Americans it read:

> For women, allow 100 lbs for the first 5 feet and 5 lbs for each additional inch. For men, allow 110 lbs for the first 5 feet and 5 lbs for each additional inch.

Broca's Index was quickly established on both sides of the Atlantic and defined healthy weight for three-quarters of a century.

By the mid-twentieth century, another industry had grown interested in our longevity—albeit for reasons a long way from medicine. In 1943, the Metropolitan Life Insurance Company decided to construct objective norms by calculating the weights associated with the lowest death rates among holders of their insurance policies. As with Broca's Index, Met Life desirable weights were lower for women than men at every height but they also distinguished between small, medium and large frames.

Met Life had a precise way of determining frame size—by wrist circumference.[26] Their frame distinction did indeed correlate with how much of excess weight was excess fat—the latter accounting for most health risk factors. However, people found measuring too complicated. Physicians ended up assessing frame by visual estimation. Patients assessed it by wishful thinking—

only 25 percent of Met Life policyholders were measured as having heavy frames, while almost all overweight patients put themselves in this category.

There was another problem with the Met Life tables: if they were used as recommended weights, they erred in the direction of being too high. This is because their data included smokers and people diagnosed with cancer soon after their weights were recorded. In making predictions from weight, which is of course the purpose for the insurance company, it's fine to combine weights low enough to *cause* disease with low weights *resulting from* disease. But if one is making recommendations, which is what everyone else immediately co-opted the Met Life tables to do, it's crucial to distinguish these. Smoking, on average, keeps weight eight pounds lower while costing twelve years of life. Undetected stomach and intestinal cancers often cause recent, unexplained weight loss. With such patients averaged in, the tables' optimal weights are somewhat higher than those that actually cause the least disease and death.

Still, the tables were more objective than previous systems and were the standard for assessing weight from the 1950s through 1980s. America's weight slowly increased, and more women than men were overweight according to the Met Life tables. Then, in the late 1980s, European medicine decided that formulas were simpler than tables and came up with the body mass index (BMI), which was very simple in the metric system:

$$BMI = \frac{\text{Weight (in kilograms)}}{\text{Height (in meters)}^2}$$

In pounds and inches it was not so easy:

$$BMI = \frac{\text{Weight (in pounds)} \times 703}{\text{Height (in inches)}^2}$$

American researchers therefore translated it into another table—albeit one with a single set of norms for all frame types:

Ht	MEN Frame Small	Medium	Large	Ht	WOMEN Frame Small	Medium	Large
5'6	136-142	139-151	146-154	4'11	103-113	111-123	120-134
5'7	138-145	142-154	149-158	5'0	104-115	113-126	122-137
5'8	140-148	145-157	152-172	5'1	106-118	115-129	125-140
5'9	142-151	148-160	155-176	5'2	108-121	118-132	128-143
5'10	144-154	151-163	158-180	5'3	111-124	121-135	131-147
5'11	146-157	154-166	161-184	5'4	114-127	124-138	134-151
6.0	149-160	157-170	164-188	5'5	117-130	127-141	137-155
6'1	152-164	160-174	168-192	5'6	120-133	130-144	140-159
6'2	155-168	164-178	172-197	5'7	123-136	133-147	143-167
6'3	158-172	167-182	176-202	5'8	126-139	136-150	146-170
6'4	162-176	171-187	181-207	5'9	129-142	139-153	149-170
6'5	166-180	175-192	186-212	5'10	132-145	142-156	152-173
6'6	170-185	180-198	192-218	5'11	135-148	145-159	155-176

Most previous tables and formulas set lower healthy weights for women (who have lighter bones and less muscle mass) than for men. The BMI standards did not. This was partly for simplifi-

BMI

WEIGHT (lbs.)

Ht	100	105	110	115	120	125	130	135	140	145	150	155	160	165	170	175	180	185	190	195	200	205	210	215	220	225	230	235	240	245	250
5'0"	20	21	21	22	23	24	25	26	27	28	29	30	31	32	33	34	35	36	37	38	39	40	41	42	43	44	45	46	47	48	49
5'1"	19	20	21	22	23	24	25	26	26	27	28	29	30	31	32	33	34	35	36	37	38	39	40	41	42	43	43	44	45	46	47
5'2"	18	19	20	21	22	23	24	25	26	27	27	28	29	30	31	32	33	34	35	36	37	37	38	39	40	41	42	43	44	45	46
5'3"	18	19	19	20	21	22	23	24	25	26	27	27	28	29	30	31	32	33	34	35	35	36	37	38	39	40	41	42	43	43	44
5'4"	17	18	19	20	21	21	22	23	24	25	26	27	27	28	29	30	31	32	33	33	34	35	36	37	38	39	39	40	41	42	43
5'5"	17	17	18	19	20	21	22	22	23	24	25	26	27	27	28	29	30	31	32	32	33	34	35	36	37	37	38	39	40	41	42
5'6"	16	17	18	19	19	20	21	22	23	23	24	25	26	27	27	28	29	30	31	31	32	33	34	35	36	36	37	38	39	40	40
5'7"	16	16	17	18	19	20	20	21	22	23	23	24	25	26	27	27	28	29	30	31	31	32	33	34	34	35	36	37	38	38	39
5'8"	15	16	17	17	18	19	20	21	21	22	23	24	24	25	26	27	27	28	29	30	30	31	32	33	33	34	35	36	36	37	38
5'9"	15	16	16	17	18	18	19	20	21	21	22	23	24	24	25	26	27	27	28	29	30	30	31	32	32	33	34	35	35	36	37
5'10"	14	15	16	17	17	18	19	19	20	21	22	22	23	24	24	25	26	27	27	28	29	29	30	31	32	32	33	34	34	35	36
5'11"	14	15	15	16	17	17	18	19	20	20	21	22	22	23	24	24	25	26	26	27	28	29	29	30	31	31	32	33	33	34	35
6'0"	14	14	15	16	16	17	18	18	19	20	20	21	22	22	23	24	24	25	26	26	27	28	28	29	30	31	31	32	33	33	34
6'1"	13	14	15	15	16	16	17	18	18	19	20	20	21	22	22	23	24	24	25	26	26	27	28	28	29	30	30	31	32	32	33
6'2"	13	13	14	15	15	16	17	17	18	19	19	20	21	21	22	22	23	24	24	25	26	26	27	28	28	29	30	30	31	31	32
6'3"	12	13	13	14	15	16	16	17	17	18	18	19	20	20	21	22	22	23	24	24	25	26	26	27	28	29	29	30	31	31	31
6'4"	12	13	13	14	15	15	16	16	17	18	18	19	19	20	21	21	22	23	23	24	24	25	26	26	27	27	28	29	29	30	30

cation and partly an attempt not to "discriminate" against women, who were categorized as obese more often than men under the Met Life norms. However, they are probably not doing women any favors with this artificial adjustment toward less obesity.

A lower BMI emerges as healthiest in recent studies that—unlike the Met Life research—exclude people who are thin from smoking and/or developing cancers. The Nurses' Health Study[27]—one of the largest medical projects ever—followed over 100,000 women thirty to fifty-five years of age for two decades, noting major illnesses and deaths and correlating them with BMI. By 1995, they had documented almost 5,000 deaths, of which slightly over half were from cancer and almost one-quarter were from cardiovascular disease. In analyses adjusted only for age, they observed a J-shaped relation between BMI and overall deaths. In other words, the thinnest women had some increased risk of dying, though not as great as the heaviest. But when smokers were excluded, there was no longer any increased risk for leaner women; risk of death rose for BMI of 19 and up. Remember, 19 is at the extreme low end of the current US and WHO "healthy" ranges. So the first category is largely people *below* recommended weight and the next two lines are people within it:

Risk of Death from All Causes

BMI	relative risk
< 19.0	1.0
19.0 to 21.9	1.2
22.0 to 24.9	1.2
25.0 to 26.9	1.3
27.0 to 28.9	1.6
29.0 to 31.9	2.1
32.0 or <	2.2

In 2001, researchers following a different group of both men and women for ten years published findings in the *Archives of Internal Medicine*[28] showing that a higher BMI increased the risk of developing common chronic diseases—again, even at some levels approved as healthy by the WHO and the US government. They concluded: "The . . . relationship between BMI and the risk of developing chronic diseases was evident even among adults in the upper half of the 'healthy' weight range (i.e., BMI of 22.0–24.9), suggesting that adults should try to maintain a BMI between 18.5 and 21.9 to minimize their risk of disease."

Results are similar in other countries and ethnic groups. A Japanese study of deaths in middle age initially found the same kind of J-shaped curve before analyzing specific patterns.[29] The deaths in the heaviest 25 percent of BMI were due primarily to coronary heart disease which is directly related to BMI. In the thinnest 25 percent, mortality was more often due to cancer and unspecified causes and was *confined to men who had lost weight between age twenty-five and examination*—not to other low BMI men. They concluded that excess deaths in thin middle-aged men were due completely to undiagnosed causes of recent weight loss, not to leanness itself: "When BMI at age twenty-five was considered, men in the bottom quintile had the lowest mortality in middle age."

Just this year, a study of diabetes among Australian aborigines found that the incidence of disease was four times greater for people with BMIs of 22 or more. Even in the 22–25 BMI range, the upper half of supposedly "normal" weight, the risk of diabetes was already close to three times greater. "We calculated that if we could prevent gains in BMI beyond 22, we could prevent an estimated 46 percent of diabetes cases . . . which is just astounding," remarked their lead researcher.[30]

These studies show that a BMI below 19 for women—pretty much the actress/Miss America norm—and a bit higher for men are those at which people are the healthiest and live the longest.

Destined to Be Fat?

The Pima Indians of Arizona are often pointed to as evidence that there are genes for obesity—and perhaps for type-2 diabetes. The Pimas have an average BMI of 30.8 for men and 35.5 for women. A BMI of 30 is the cutoff for obesity, so the *average* Pima is obese—69 percent actually fall into this range. The prevalence of full-blown type-2 diabetes is 54 percent for men and 32 percent for women.[31] The Arizona Pimas live a sedentary lifestyle, and eat lots of highly processed, high-calorie, low-nutrition foods. However, researchers find that they live similarly to many Native American tribes who are heavier on average than whites but still much lighter than the Pimas.

The Pimas inspired the "thrifty gene" hypothesis— that some peoples evolved a tendency to put on fat more efficiently than others. After comparing Pimas to other Americans, some researchers estimate that 40–70 percent of variance of body fat can be ascribed to genetics.[32] Photos of the outsized tribe lingering in diabetes clinics became the obligatory example when arguing that obesity was genetic.

There's much truth to this. Humans obviously have developed an ability to store fat—and some subgroups do so more efficiently than others. But Pimas are not destined to be obese. Looking at modern individuals, it's easy to believe this. But it is completely wrong. No trait is ever so genetic as to exclude interaction with the environment. Researchers began to notice some Pimas had tintypes of their grandparents—and these people weren't particularly overweight. Then they noticed an even more interesting group of thin Pimas.

About seven hundred years ago, the Pima tribe separated into two geographic locations: Arizona and the Sierra Madre mountains of Mexico. That isn't enough time for them to diverge genetically, but it's plenty of time for eating and exercise patterns to change. The Mexican Pimas practice traditional, non-mechanized farming. On the steep slopes, they cultivate corn and beans as their main staples plus seasonal vegetables and fruits such as zucchini squash, tomatoes, garlic, green pepper, peaches and apples. They also gather wild plants. They mill lumber—by hand. There is no electricity or running water in their homes, and they walk long distances for water to drink and to wash their clothes. They use no modern devices for grinding cornmeal or any other household chores.

Mexican Pimas average twenty-three hours of hard physical labor a week. Arizona Pimas get less than five hours of any exercise. The Mexican Pimas eat a diet lower in fat and refined carbohydrates than the Arizona Pimas—or than most Americans. The Mexican Pimas on average weigh sixty-five pounds less than Arizona Pimas. Their average BMI is about 25 for both men and women—less than the average American. Their rate of diabetes is 10 percent for women and 6 percent for men.[33]

The poverty of the Arizona Pimas was sometimes cited as another factor in their obesity; but Mexican Pimas are poorer still. That is, unless one thinks in terms of Lee and DeVore's concept of "affluent" hunter-gatherers: then the Mexican Pimas are somewhat affluent in terms of their available foods, but, like most groups that practice agriculture, they have a poverty of leisure time.

How Good Is the BMI? A Lesson in Lilliputian Physics

All these studies I've been citing on health and weight use the BMI as their measure, so you might assume it's the most scientific method of assessing a person's best weight. Oddly, this is not the case.

Not only would the BMI be better if the norms were adjusted

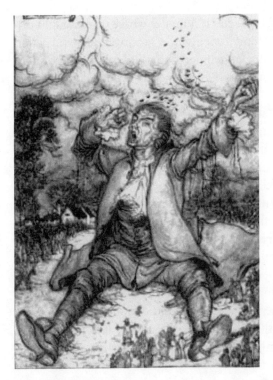

Gulliver meets
the Lilliputians.
(Courtesy of the
Estate of Arthur
Rackham. Bridgeman
Art Library)

downward and distinguished by gender, but replacing it with a
very different formula would be best of all. Proportions can't tell
us enough about body composition and, as I'll say more about in
a minute, measures of muscle-to-fat ratio are preferable. Less
obviously to many people, BMI doesn't really measure even
body proportions accurately. I've had more than one physician
argue with me until they review their junior high geometry
slowly, so it's worth examining this point a bit—especially if
you're unusually tall or short.

The basic flaw in the BMI formula is that the denominator
of height is only squared, which means that a short person will
have a lower BMI than a tall person with the same body shape.

The BMI's "ideal" is based on a model where one should keep the exact same circumference while getting taller and taller. It's a fundamental law of geometry that volume, and therefore mass and weight, increase by the product of *three* dimensions, not by two.

The best illustration of this I've seen is one Randy Schellenberg uses in writing about anorexia nervosa.[34] Schellenberg applies BMI calculations to Jonathan Swift's fantasy novel *Gulliver's Travels*, in which Gulliver encountered two strange races of people: the tiny Lilliputians and the giant Brobdingnagians. The Brobdingnagians were proportioned like Gulliver but were ten times his height, while the Lilliputians were one-tenth his height. In reality the Brobdingnagians couldn't exist, because of the engineering principle that as something increases in size, it must be made of stronger materials to support the same proportions. Lilliputians would run into the problem that some proportions would dictate membranes less than one cell-width thick. People already exist in pretty much the whole size range our design allows. However, the imaginary Lilliputians and Brobdingnagians make an excellent illustration of what's wrong with the squaring of height in the BMI formula.

If Gulliver was six feet tall and weighed 180 pounds, his BMI would be near the top of the WHO-US "normal" range:

$$[\ 180 \ / \ (72 \times 72) \ ] \times 703 = 24.4$$

A typical Brobdingnagian, however, if proportioned identically, would weigh 180,000 pounds—because if he's ten times taller, then he's also ten times wider and ten times deeper front-to-back, or $10 \times 10 \times 10 = 1{,}000$ times the weight. He would have a BMI of:

$$[\ 180{,}000 \ / \ (720 \times 720) \ ] \times 703 = 244$$

A typical Lilliputian would weigh only .18 pound and would have a BMI of:

$$[0.18 / (7.2 \times 7.2)] \times 703 = 2.44$$

These extreme examples may seem ridiculous and irrelevant, but let's scale Gulliver up by 19 percent to 7'2", the tall end of the range for NBA basketball players. In order to keep the same proportions, he would weigh 306 pounds and would have a BMI of:

$$[306 / (86 \times 86)] \times 703 = 29.1$$

He would now be technically classified as obese. Now let's scale Gulliver down from his 6' size to 4'2". He would now weigh 60 pounds and have a BMI well below the "normal" range:

$$[60 / (50 \times 50)] \times 703 = 16.9$$

The most desirable proportions for a human may not stay exactly the same across all heights—some body organs such as the brain are only slightly smaller in a short person than a taller one. And it's not that BMI should be cubing height; only in a cube-shaped object is the volume found that way. Taking height and not depth and width is arbitrary also—but then amplifying it in two rather than three dimensions doesn't correct that. There are two geometric confounds that work reasonably well only because humans come in such a narrow range of heights.

All Pounds Are Not Created Equal

"Fat thin person" is a term I first heard from my colleague Arreed Barabasz, in co-teaching hypnosis and fitness workshops. Arreed is one of the psychologists-who-became-personal-trainers that I mentioned in Chapter 4. His pet phrase is not an oxymoron—it accurately describes an increasingly common physique. If you limit calories but those calories are non-nutritious and you don't exercise, you're likely to have low muscle mass, deposits of fat and yet a "healthy" BMI. The "fat thin person" highlights that the much maligned term "fat" is actually the most accurate one. Athletes can, in some sense, be "heavy" or "overweight" but not "fat." The accumulation of excess adipose cells is what's unhealthy—and this can begin at relatively low weights.

Even if BMI treated us as three-dimensional objects rather than two-dimensional ones, it still wouldn't tell us what that body mass consists of. As common sense would suggest, the percentage of our weight that is fat turns out to be a stronger health predictor than any weight-to-height ratio.[35] When we look at body fat percentage, we exclude muscle, bone, brain and other organs which aren't supposed to be smaller for health. For some diseases, such as cardiovascular ones, body fat percentage predicts risk twice as well as BMI. Studies that specifically examine deep abdominal body fat percentage yield even better predictions of health and longevity, as this type of fat seems to be more involved with biochemical processes that stimulate cancer growth and cardiovascular damage.[36]

The main reason body fat percentage is not used in most studies is that it is more difficult and expensive to measure than BMI. The best test is the dual energy X-ray absorptiometry, or DEXA—and this is the only one that can assess deep abdominal fat versus subcutaneous fat. Other measures of body fat, in decreasing order of accuracy, are: underwater weight displacement, in which one is submerged in a large tank of water and must exhale all air from the lungs for the moment of assessment; electrical impedance tests, in which a very mild electrical current is passed through the body (some home scales now have a crude version of this); and calipers, which pinch the skin (they actually measure the less important kind of fat—subcutaneous—though for most people it correlates somewhat with their deeper fat). Arreed and many trainers these days have people get an accurate body fat assessment at the start of their work to provide a basis for tracking progress.

Body Fat Percentages[37]

	Men	Women
Average American	22%	32%
Healthy Americans	12–18%	19–25%
Hunter-Gatherers	5–15%	20–25%
Top Athletes	3–12%	10–18%

There are other measures besides body fat percentage which correlate with health better than BMI. One is waist-to-hip ratio; this measure has been found to predict both heart disease and cancer better than BMI.[38] It is interesting to note that waist–to-hip ratio also predicts aesthetic ratings of the female body better than BMI. Even the simpler measure of absolute waist measurement, without factoring in height or hip girth, predicts type-2 diabetes and heart disease more accurately than BMI.[39]

So why does BMI work even as well as it does? All these measures correlate somewhat with one another—especially at the lower end of their ranges. Whereas it's possible to have an unusually muscular person with a very high BMI, it's almost impossible to have someone in the most desirable BMI range of 18–20 without a low body fat percentage, low waist-to-hip ratio and small waist size. Large muscles are rare in our culture, and people over 6'6" and under 5' are few. Still, I'd encourage researchers to use body fat percentage or even just waist measurement instead of BMI. But for the purpose of summarizing existing research, I'm going to keep quoting BMI findings through the rest of this book.

Calorie-Restriction Research

An even more dramatic body of research is emerging on "calorie restriction" or CR. For almost a century, evidence has been building that—if vitamins, protein and other trace nutrients are well-supplied—dropping calories far below that needed to maintain normal weight results in up to a 65 percent longer lifespan, with more activity and better health, for a variety of animals ranging from worms to mammals. Primate studies—and, recently, ones in humans—are finding that health improves and aging slows on this regimen. Researchers go so far as to suggest that this points to a human lifespan of 120 to 150 years and to an optimal BMI even lower than 19.

Calorie-restriction research began in 1914, when Francis

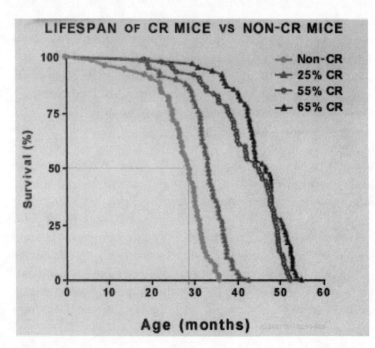

Peyton Rous (who later received a Nobel Prize for cancer research) published a study showing that reduced food intake lowered the rate of tumors in rodents.[40] In 1917, distinguished Yale nutritionists Osborne and Mendel published findings in *Science* that rats on low-calorie diets lived longer and were fertile at a later age.[41]

Over the next several decades, these findings were repeated in yeast, worms, flies, spiders, fish and several types of rodents—with lifespan increases varying from 25 to 65 percent, depending on degree and length of CR.[42] Consistently, CR animals were healthier throughout their lives. In 2002, the first study of a longer-lived large mammal was completed. Golden retrievers with calories restricted by 25 percent lived a year and a half longer than their free-feeding littermates. The most common medical problem for this breed—hip arthritis—was delayed in onset by three years.[43]

In the 1970s, Roy Walford and his colleagues at UCLA began to focus on discovering the mechanism(s) by which CR slowed aging. They found stronger immune-system responsiveness in older calorie-restricted mice, enhanced DNA repair, more efficient function of the mitochondria or energy centers of the cell, and lower average body temperature—the latter likely to reduce metabolic stress on the organism.[44]

Most of the CR research restricted calories since weaning—virtually all of an animal's life. This is not anything humans are likely to want to imitate. However, Walford's group quickly established that caloric restriction worked when it was initiated in mice at twelve months (early middle age), though the lifespan extension was less dramatic than when initiated with pups. Very recently, Stephen R. Spindler of the University of California, Riverside, has found that CR works even in old age. Nineteen-month-old mice, about the human equivalent of sixty to sixty-five years, lived up to six months longer if switched to fewer calories.

Spindler found that restricting calories for old mice immediately slowed measures of aging. The dietary change added about 42 percent to the remaining lifespan of the calorie-restricted mice.[45] This appears to be a fairly consistent formula across species: restricting calories by 25 percent extends lifespan by 25 percent of what would otherwise be the remaining years from the point at which it is begun, 40 percent restriction increases by 40 percent the remaining years . . . up to about 50 percent restriction.

Monkeys are among our closest relatives; in the late 1980s and early 1990s three primate studies began—two in rhesus monkeys and one in squirrel monkeys. Even without CR, they live at least twenty years, so there is not yet complete longevity data. However, the CR monkeys do manifest many of the age-delaying benefits found in lower animals such as lower blood lipids, better insulin and glucose metabolism and heightened immune function. There is already a trend toward more die-off in the free-feeding groups than in the CR ones. One of the underfed monkeys is already thirty-eight years old, the human equivalent of 114, though final data won't be in for a decade.[46]

"We *don't want* flies to live longer!"
—Longevity researcher Robert Arking's
future mother-in-law, when told
what he did for a living.[47]

No studies of human calorie restriction have yet lasted long enough to measure lifespan. However, it is no longer preposterous for researchers to state that animal extrapolations imply human equivalents of 120 to 150 years. Two shorter-term human studies have already reported health results much like the monkey data.

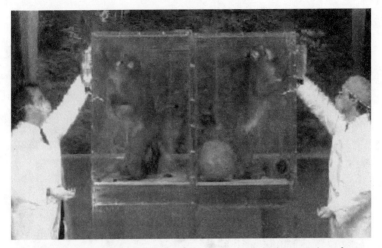

The calorie-restricted monkey on the left is smaller, has a higher muscle-to-fat ratio, is more active and shows many fewer signs of aging than his free-feeding counterpart on the right. *(Photo courtesy of National Institutes of Health, Bethesda, Maryland)*

In 1991, eight people were selected from among hundreds of applicants to be sealed inside the Biosphere 2—a futuristic glass structure in the Arizona desert. This was originally intended as an exercise in environmental self-sufficiency, not as a dietary experiment. At the outset, only one person followed a calorie-restricted regimen: the directors of Biosphere had specified that one occupant needed to be a physician, and Dr. Walford of the long-lived mice was selected.

In the first months of Biosphere 2, it was discovered that the dome would be unable to grow as much food as projected and importing produce would compromise its self-sufficiency. Walford proposed that everyone reduce food consumption by 25 percent while taking vitamin and mineral supplements. The crew agreed and a fortuitous study began. During the first six months, the Biospherians' weight dropped from an average of 163 to 137 pounds for the men and from 134 to 119 for

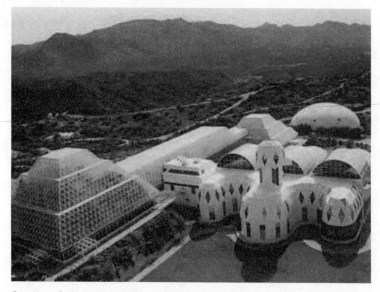

Biosphere 2. (© *Jan Butchofsky-Houser / Corbis*)

the women. Their blood pressure dropped from 109/74 to 89/58 and their serum cholesterol levels decreased by 35 percent. Glucose metabolism, lymphocyte and neutrophil function all improved.[48]

The Biosphere study was extraordinarily well controlled. It's rare that you have human research where you can be sure your subjects aren't sneaking off to McDonald's at least once during the study, or that they all report on time for every physiological measurement. The drawbacks were that Biosphere was shorter-term and involved fewer people than would be ideal.

In 2006, the *Journal of the American Medical Association* published a small but well-controlled study of a group of overweight but non-obese people who reduced their calories by 25 percent while still eating optimally nutritionally.[49] They showed not only changes associated with better health, such as improved insulin metabolism, but also ones associated with less aging, such as less DNA damage in cells. They did not start off at normal weight or achieve extreme thinness, so their absolute health parameters were not as impressive as those of the Biosphere participants during the short experiment.

There is a group of people who have followed a CR diet longer than the Biospherians or the *JAMA* subjects. This is the Calorie Restriction Society—a loose confederation of individuals interested in CR research and translating it into their own health. They are scattered all over the globe and don't eat exactly the same diet; their "groupness" consists simply of a shared interest in applying the results of CR research to their own lives. There is no universally agreed-upon translation from animal research to human meals, although Roy Walford offered his suggestions in the 1991 book *The 120 Year Diet* and two current leaders of the CR Society followed up with the 2005 *Longevity Diet*.[50] Most CR Society members reduce their calories by 10 to 40 percent and eat lean protein, lots of fresh vegetables, some fruit and whole grains. Many also take supplements containing vitamins, minerals and antioxidants.

CRS members stay in touch via a website[51] with elaborate discussion groups—and, for some of them, an annual conference. I went to the 2006 meeting. It was easy to pick out who was attending CRS versus other events in the lobby of an Arizona hotel. Most members are thin, some extremely gaunt. Lisa Walford has a BMI of 15. That's less than fashion models and, indeed, she probably looks a bit too thin by aesthetic ideals. However, she's obviously in great health after decades on this diet. She led yoga sessions at the conference, which she does for a living, and she radiated vitality and energy. In general, members seemed healthy and some looked quite a bit younger than their stated ages. (Asking someone's age is more acceptable in this group than most.)

The CRS meeting had successfully persuaded the hotel to

feed us nothing even resembling hotel food. Every meal was a buffet with huge bowls of baby spinach, dark lettuces, other greens and chopped vegetables. There was always some form of protein—fish or chicken—ground into small pieces to sprinkle on as a garnish. There was a choice of olive oil or calorie-free dressing. And fruit. Most of the diners skipped any dressing. Some skipped the fruit. Others were on more specific regimens and brought various sprouts or protein powders. Some were fasting entirely on one or more days. I found it remarkably easy to stay with their diet when sitting in a room with only those selections. It was an odd reversal of my usual role to be the most indulgent person in line by virtue of sprinkling olive oil over my salad.

CRS members seemed to be having as good a time at meals as anyone else. Some were clearly enjoying the food per se, others didn't pay much attention to their food but engaged in animated conversation. Most told me that the diet had been difficult at first and that they'd initially felt hungry, but that these problems had disappeared over time. A few mentioned ongoing daily bouts of hunger but still believed the regimen was worthwhile for its benefits in health and energy. Several said they'd been on more extreme versions of CR which made them tired, depressed or irritable until they restored a small percentage of calories. A tendency to get chilly more easily was the one common side effect many of them mentioned.

A young physician, Luigi Fontana, has undertaken to study this group. He published the first findings in 2005, based on members of the group who had followed various degrees of CR for at least six years.[52] Their current health test results were compared to their medical records before beginning the diet. The CRS members showed major improvements in all the parameters from the Biosphere study and also on additional ones of muscle-to-fat ratio, insulin responsiveness and carotid artery thickness—all measures of improved health and youthfulness. Fontana and his team did not hazard any specific predictions about lifespan for the group, but he did conclude, "Our research has shown that a chronic reduction of calorie intake exerts a potent protective effect against some of the illnesses that are the principal causes of death and disability in industrialized countries. It is certain that the prospects for the people involved in the investigation are better than the average, as most likely they will not suffer blocking of the arteries, diabetes or arterial hypertension, conditions that cause, frequently, heart attacks and strokes." At the meeting I attended, Fontana presented his data on markers for cancer risk, which looked equally positive.[53]

Some CR researchers are looking not just at *whether* CR extends life and health, but *how* it does so. Its direct effects— lower body fat, lower blood pressure and better glucose and insulin metabolism—are likely to produce a longer average lifespan. However, animal experiments also extended *maximal* lifespan—the longest any member of a species has been recorded to live—so metabolic changes which could account for this have been examined. CR lowers the creation of free radicals and glycolated proteins, the two substances most linked to age-related damage to cells. It activates the sirtuin family of proteins, which exist in both plants and animals as a mechanism to help them survive famines. All three of these mechanisms are being pursued by pharmaceutical companies looking for chemicals to mimic each aspect of calorie restriction—but for now, the most powerful way to achieve them is to really restrict calories.

Okinawa

By now you may be wondering why there aren't any people living to record-setting ages from among underfed areas or periods of history. However, all the animal research and the Biosphere and CR Society studies involve dropping calories while carefully supplementing vitamins, minerals and protein. All extremely calorie-depriving situations throughout history, such as famine and concentration camps, involved major deprivation of nutrients as well. Even in terms of milder, voluntary diets, until very recently supplements didn't exist and fruits and vegetables were not shipped across the world year round.

The closest thing to a naturalistic version of CR is the Japanese district of Okinawa. Here diet consists of a higher percentage of fresh vegetables than in most places, and fish and soy make up virtually all the protein. Okinawans eat some rice but less than on mainland Japan. Most importantly, Okinawans explicitly teach their children that it is healthy to get up from the table a bit hungry. Adults consume 40 percent fewer calories than Americans and 17 percent fewer calories than the Japanese average. The caloric intake of Okinawan children is 36 percent below the Japanese *recommended intake*. This is not as extreme as animal studies and most Okinawans are not taking the supplements that CR Society people do. However, it's the closest to a naturalist version of a calorie-restricted, nutrient-adequate diet anywhere.

Okinawa has the longest average lifespan in the world and the highest percentage of centenarians (people living to one hundred or more).[54] Not only do Okinawans have reduced mortality, but, also consistent with animal CR research, they enjoy reduced morbidity from a range of causes. Compared to Americans, Okinawan elders:

- are 75 percent more likely to retain cognitive ability
- get 80 percent fewer breast and prostate cancers
- get 50 percent fewer ovarian and colon cancers
- have 50 percent fewer hip fractures
- have 80 percent fewer heart attacks

So what's too thin? I'll leave the question of whether one can be too rich to personal taste, and obviously there's *some* weight that's too thin—but it's far more extreme than we often think. A BMI of 12–12.5 corresponds to the point at which humans die of starvation. At a BMI of 13–15 most people are ill—chilly, tired and often with depressed immune systems or wasting of heart muscle or other organ tissue. As I mentioned, Lisa Walford reports a BMI of 15 but she's also a very short woman (remember your Lilliputian physics), so most may need a slightly higher BMI for good health; at the CR meeting, most of the women who'd ever dropped below 16 or men beneath 17.5 seemed to have not felt their best at these weights. The Met Life tables were right on two counts: people's frames vary, and on average men should probably be a bit heavier than women because they average more muscle mass for a given height.

People See Weight Problems Everywhere but in the Mirror

A 2006 Pew poll found that most Americans think that their fellow citizens are overweight, but they're slow to realize that they themselves might be. The chart below—based on polling 2,250 absolutely average adults, not the unusually slim—shows how perceptions vary between the way people view the public versus friends versus self. In the poll, respondents also underestimated their own weight (women more than men), and overestimated their height (men more than women). They tended to classify themselves as "exercising moderately" when they did next to nothing and as eating "moderately healthy" on a diet of mostly high-fat, high-sugar, excess-calorie foods. Though 45 percent were "trying to lose weight" (tellingly more than said they were overweight), this is a lower

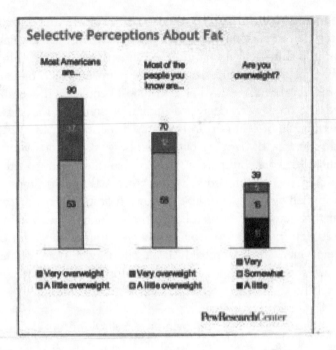

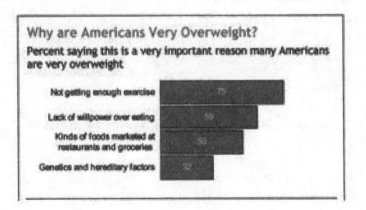

number than a decade ago. Most rated dieting as "very hard" and were not successful at it.

The poll also asked *why* people are overweight. Seventy per cent believed inadequate exercise was very significant, 59 percent said lack of willpower about what to eat, 50 percent attributed it to the kinds of foods marketed at restaurants and grocery stores, and 32 percent chose genetics and hereditary factors. It might be encouraging that individual efforts such as exercise and willpower are seen as more important than external ones such as menus and genetics—except that these respondents are talking about other people, remember. Their explanations about themselves are . . . well . . . they're *not* overweight, so they don't explain *why* they're overweight. Also the poll presents false dichotomies: foods versus genetics, menus versus willpower. Of course the cause is an interaction between these things. We need to approach the problem from all angles. Chapter 8 will discuss approaches to aid willpower about food and exercise, while the final chapter will discuss how we can get the wrong foods off our grocery shelves and restaurant menus.

8

Marching to a Different Drummer: Strategies for the Individual in an Unhealthy Society

So what can we do within our current environment to get or stay healthy? I'll summarize the practical implications of previous chapters briefly because they're important but very simple. *How* to make such changes is the difficult part and will occupy most of this chapter.

In terms of diet, people should eat lots of dark, fibrous vegetables, moderate amounts of lean protein and fruits, and small servings of nuts, other seeds (including grains) and eggs. No one should eat *any* trans fats, white flour or refined sugar. Those who are overweight need to eat fewer calories—there's no universal number: just drop calories till you're losing weight. Exercise at least an hour a day.

For readers who want more detail, there exist a number of sound diet books. *The Paleo Diet*, *The Paleolithic Prescription* and *NeanderThin* focus on recreating what our hunter-gatherer ancestors ate.[1] *The 120 Year Diet* and *The Longevity Diet* describe the use of calorie restriction to extend lifespan. Any book with "macrobiotic" in the title suggests how to eat food at its freshest to maximize nutrients. And finally, *The Perricone Prescription*[2] has its quirky origin with a dermatologist seeking foods to delay wrinkles. Even though these books begin from different premises, they all converge on similar food lists and recipes elaborating on fresh unprocessed foods.

I don't, however, particularly recommend this amount of attention to eating plans and recipes. Complicating diets can increase procrastination and derail people from changing their eating habits. If I were writing a recipe book, the entries would look like the box below. Food doesn't need extensive preparation to be healthy. Supernormal stimuli take more time than healthy meals.

Spinach and Tuna Salad

Place half a bag of pre-washed baby spinach into a bowl. Open an 8 oz. can of water-packed tuna, drain, dump over spinach.

Tofu with Asian Vegetables

Chop tofu, mushrooms, broccoli, red bell peppers and/or mung sprouts. Place these in a wok or ordinary skillet with 1 tbsp. canola oil. Add soy sauce. Or not. Stir occasionally over medium heat while talking on phone or testing whether your cat will eat tofu. After 4–10 minutes, serve.

Take-out Fast Food

Enter convenience store or grocery.
Locate small box of raisins and small bag of raw walnuts.
Go to cashier—lines shorter than at burger chains.

The idea that fast-food restaurants, TV dinners and packaged "instant" or "quick" meals save us from some enormous time-sink involved in preparing food is a ploy advertisers have repeated so often that we've come to accept it. But it's ludicrous. Only ingredients people shouldn't be eating anyway—refined fats, flour, granulated sugar—take time to convert back into something resembling food. Chopping whole foods to eat raw or steamed doesn't take long at all.

If you're slim and fit and enjoy preparing elaborate recipes from a rich array of healthy, natural ingredients, by all means practice this form of self-expression. However, it isn't necessary to go to that much trouble to avoid unhealthy junk food.

And—though this is more difficult to accept—if you're trying to lose weight, you might reconsider whether maximizing the tastiness of your food should really be a goal. Through most of history, adding sugar, oils or elaborate seasoning was something done to coax the very ill or elderly who'd lost normal hunger to eat. Everyone else was expected to consume what was at hand. Now almost all our meals resemble what we would serve an emaciated invalid.

Stay away from the supernormal stimuli—that's what tastes the very best. Eat natural foods, even though they may at first seem boring to long-overstimulated palates. If you feel like eating less of them—*that's part of the point*. In Tinbergen's bird experiments, if he tried to remove the giant Day-Glo, polka-dot plaster egg, the bird would fight to keep it, then hunt for it a while, but eventually resume a normal response to its own tiny, bluish, grey-dappled eggs. It's only when supernormal stimuli are present or have just been removed that eating real food seems like a deprivation. Once you avoid the supernormal stimuli, natural foods begin to taste as good to you as they did to your ancestors.

Let's return for a minute to the analogy of drug addiction. Supernormal stimuli have instinctual appeal at first glance. Our modern junk food has this going for it—plus a reinforced biological response after repeated glucose peaks. We all hear people talk about how they couldn't possibly give up cheeseburgers and fries entirely, or that it's cruel or unreasonable to suggest they never eat dessert. But as a psychologist, I hear from addicts how completely unimaginable never shooting up again seems or how they just couldn't get through the day without a certain number of drinks or pills. Both are compellingly heartfelt but just not accurate. When you begin to eat healthily, within days, glucose and hunger-regulating hormones shift, diminishing cravings. Within weeks, a positive conditioned response becomes associated with fish or spinach and extinguishes to French fries or mousse. If fresh vegetables or steamed fish don't appeal to you in a couple of weeks, this will mean *you're not hungry*.

The loss of years incurred by heroin use per se (as opposed to illegal supplies and reused needles) is not even as much as for morbid obesity.[3] However, the time when heroin and cocaine were sold in over-the-counter health tonics is so long past that it may be difficult for the modern reader to see these as equivalents. Perhaps the better analogy is tobacco. Within the lifetime of half my readers, cigarette smoking was such a socially approved pleasure that asking the person next to you in a restaurant or plane not to smoke was outrageous. Yet tobacco was already known to be a deadly health risk—that fact just oddly coexisted with its innocuous image. The last chapter will address how we can alter the similarly wholesome image of deadly eating habits at the broad societal level. But in the remainder of this chapter, we'll look at altering it within the microcosm of our own attitudes and behavior.

Psychology Can Help—But Maybe Not in the Way You've Been Told

Martin Seligman, founder of the field of Positive Psychology, begins his book *What You Can Change and What You Can't* with the following vignette:

Trudy weighed 175 pounds when she graduated from Brown a decade ago. Four times since, she has slimmed down to under 125: Weight Watchers, Nutri-System, six months under the care of a private behavior therapist, and last year, Optifast. With each regime the weight came off quickly, if not painlessly. Each time, the fat returned, faster and more of it. Trudy now weighs 195 and has given up.

Seligman uses the vignette to set up the central question he's addressing in his book:

What can we succeed in changing about ourselves? What can we not? Why did Trudy fail? . . . When can we overcome our biology? When is our biology our destiny?

He proceeds to answer this question by telling us that panic disorder and sexual dysfunction can both be "easily unlearned," that "our moods are readily controlled" and that "depression can be cured." However, Seligman says, "Dieting, in the long run, almost never works."[4]

This isn't the disingenuous cliché of many diet books that quickly define dieting in a narrow sense of temporarily altering one's diet in a radical manner. Those diet books cast other diets as advocating this (virtually none do) and offer themselves as the main proponent for altering one's eating sensibly for a lifetime. Seligman isn't playing that semantic game; he means what "dieting" *really* means: any attempt to reduce weight by altering what we eat—including moderate, lifetime plans. *This* is what he's telling us almost never works. Seligman doesn't go into much detail about why it doesn't work; he just says it's because of "biology." He's writing a book on self-acceptance and happiness, after all, not weight or fitness. Seligman's point is that Trudy would be happier if she accepted that she is destined to

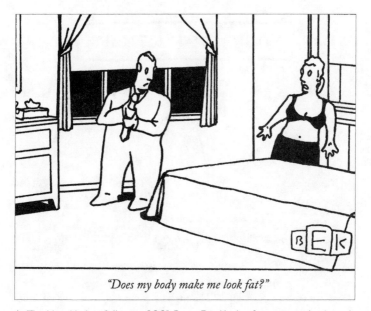

"Does my body make me look fat?"

remain overweight: "Much of successful living consists of learning to make the best of a bad situation."

So what are we to make of this advice to would-be dieters? Seligman is a major thinker in psychology, albeit not a specialist in health psychology. The suggestion that overweight people might rationally examine their options and choose to remain overweight is usually ignored, almost a taboo. It deserves serious consideration rather than being discarded out of hand, and Seligman deserves credit for being so bold as to raise it.

Looking at the research, he also has an important statistical point. "Dieting, in the long run, almost never works" is only a slight overstatement of studies which find that, despite efforts to address maintenance, maximal weight loss is typically achieved at around six months, followed by weight regain.[5] In one of the longest-term research projects, which followed patients for four

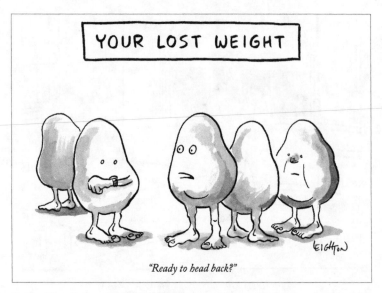

"Ready to head back?"

(© The New Yorker Collection 2003 Robert Leighton from cartoonbank.com)

to five years after their initial weight loss, *less than 3 percent* were at or below their post-treatment weight on all follow-up visits.[6] On average, the group still had some weight loss at long-term follow-up, but a negatively accelerating pattern of weight regain was the predominant outcome.

However, Seligman makes the common mistake of assuming that if someone is overweight with a fast-food, low-exercise lifestyle, this is biological destiny. This doesn't take into account the interaction of instinct with the environment; it misses what the biological implications really are.

What Psychology Can't Do

There is a vast psychological literature on why we overeat—some helpful, much of it not. I'm going to briefly review some of the approaches to avoid before turning to what research suggests does help. It is not helpful to routinely tell overweight people that their problem is caused by a neurotic need to "comfort yourself with food" or "fill an inner emptiness." It is not helpful to tell people that they will need long-term psychotherapy to understand their neuroses before they can slim down. As I've stressed throughout this book, humans have an evolutionary, biological tendency to gain weight when supplied with the sugar/salt/fat/calorie-rich, nutrient-poor modern diet—and while getting little exercise. If you're depressed or anxious—or even psychotic—this will certainly complicate a weight problem, but it's not the main cause, and it doesn't necessarily need to be resolved before successful dieting can occur. It's analogous to smoking: those who say they smoke to reduce anxiety or depression find additional challenges in giving up cigarettes but nevertheless often quit before recovering from their psychological problems.

One reason psychoanalytic-style therapy has been thought to be helpful with habit change is the placebo effect. When highly motivated people are offered an interpretation that is said to enable them to change, they sometimes do. In the 1930s, psychologist George Kelly performed an informal experiment exploring why Freudian interpretations, which he regarded as patently preposterous, sometimes led to change. He began, in his own words, "fabricating insights" and "offered preposterous interpretations" to clients. "Some of them were about as un-Freudian as I could make them." Kelly observed that to have a chance of changing behavior the "only criteria were that the explanation account for the crucial facts as the client saw them, and that it carry implications for approaching the future in a different way."[7] Cognitive-behavioral therapy has adopted the concept of shaking up thought patterns as conducive to change while discarding the fabricated insights.

The other reason psychodynamic psychotherapy sometimes helps weight loss is that, *occasionally*, someone actually is overweight for a specific psychological reason. I've seen a few patients who were so deprived in childhood that food was their only pleasure. Developing the physical and social skills to enjoy other pursuits helped them enormously in enduring the discomforts of dieting. There are some survivors of sexual abuse for whom any sexual attention makes them so anxious that obesity represents a welcome escape. Usually such people are fully aware of this motive; only occasionally is it unconscious. I once treated a survivor of childhood sexual abuse for whom obesity represented not discouraging of sexual attention but rather power. She had experienced the horror of being raped as a function of a heavier person being able to hold her down. This equation was unconscious until, during a hypnotic session exploring her weight loss plateauing at 200 pounds, a childlike subpersonality explained that she couldn't ever again weigh less than her father. This patient lost further weight only after cognitive work on understanding safety as more closely related to strength training and self-defense knowledge. Similarly, the more common fear of being attractive is addressed with social assertiveness training.

Even with these extreme examples, the causes interact with our food environment. Hunter-gatherers had their share of childhood abuse and other bad parenting, but it didn't lead to obesity. For the vast majority of people, even the initial source of their overeating isn't psychological.

What Psychology Can Do

Two areas of psychology research are most important in understanding our weight and fitness crisis: that on habit and that on self-control or willpower. We'll examine each of these briefly before moving on to which therapy techniques help break bad habits and increase self-control.

Habit. Recent brain-scanning technology has enabled us to see our habits at work. When we do something familiar without even thinking about it, an area deep within our brain—the basal ganglia—fires in an exact sequence. Thus we drive or walk our habitual route to work and arrive without a sense of having decided to make specific turns. When the route was new to us, a very different brain area—the prefrontal neocortex—lit up as we decided whether to turn left here or wondered which street had more traffic on it. This mass of gray matter just above our eyes controls the conscious weighing of complex logical decisions. It works slowly and carefully. As we learn the route, the basal ganglia begin to get involved, generating a known pattern and actually suppressing other possibilities of action. The prefrontal neocortex either quiets as we travel to work, or turns to other matters such as a task we'll start upon when we arrive or vacation plans next month.

Now if we're eating badly or not exercising, we don't want habits to continue uninterrupted. The first stage of change is to engage the prefrontal neocortex and ponder healthier options. When we begin a diet or exercise program, this area will be active with questions such as "What's the healthiest entrée on this menu?" or "Would I rather start running in the morning or join that new gym class?" or even "Do I really want to stick with this diet or would I really rather order some ice cream?" However, we don't want to stay in the frontal area indefinitely. It's effortful, and either outcome can always result. We want to make the healthy choice so consistently that our basal ganglia take over and soon we don't even weigh the new choices, we just take the healthy option: waitress approaches, order the garden vegetables; it's morning, put on running shoes. This stage of effortfully making consistent healthy choices involves another area psychology has researched.

Willpower. In many circles, willpower is almost a dirty word. Weight-loss experts like to say that overeating is "not about a lack of willpower." But all "willpower" means is deciding to do something and resolutely following through without getting derailed by short-term discomforts or temptations. Do we *really* doubt that this exists, or that it would apply to weight loss? If deciding that you are going on a diet and then ending up overeating is not a "lack of willpower," then what on earth would you call it?

The most generous interpretation of why people don't like the concept of willpower is that when so many people possess so little, it may lead them to feel bad about themselves. Even if willpower were an unchangeable trait, however, it would still be helpful to have an accurate assessment of one's own. If you're otherwise high on the ability to stick with resolutions and yet you're overweight, the first priority probably needs to be really getting serious in your conviction about the importance of changing your diet and exercise. If you're short on willpower, you might want to put more emphasis on environmental manipulations. If you don't keep rich foods in your house and decline buffet party invitations your basal ganglia can run the show more of the time and your prefrontal cortex won't be put to the test.

There's some value in the recommendations above, but it also turns out that willpower is a trainable skill. Studies find initial individual differences, but people can greatly improve their willpower through practice. Howard Rankin, who did some of the earliest research in the 1970s at the University of London, advises first visualizing the desired new habits and then gradually exposing oneself to temptation. Rankin uses the analogy of muscular exercise: "The important point is to successfully do it enough times to strengthen your willpower by flexing it."[8]

In a recent Australian study, people who hadn't taken part in any regular physical activity for at least twelve months began practicing willpower exercises designed to get them exercising regularly. Not only was this effective for motivating their exercise regime, but it generalized to other areas. During the two-month study, subjects also reported smoking less and consuming less alcohol. Healthy eating, emotional control, maintenance of household chores, adherence to commitments, monitoring of spending and good study habits increased.[9] "If you think about the over-consumption of unhealthy foods, lack of exercise, gambling and drugs, then self-control could be one of the most important medicines for our time," observed the lead author of the study.[10] When we've come to consider it reasonable, almost routine, for the obese to have part of their stomach removed to make overeating more difficult—despite a 40 percent rate of serious complications such as intestinal leakage, bowel obstruction, wound infection or nutritional deficiency[11]—it's time to think of willpower training as a viable alternative.

Psychological research has found that two techniques are the most effective in helping people to lose weight: cognitive-

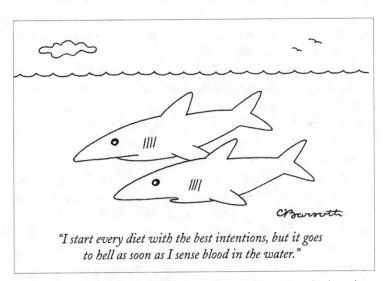

"I start every diet with the best intentions, but it goes
to hell as soon as I sense blood in the water."

(© The New Yorker Collection 1999 Charles Barsotti from cartoonbank.com)

behavioral strategies, and hypnosis/imagery/visualization.[12] These are the same two that are emphasized in general willpower enhancement, and they both serve the goal of eventually turning control over to a new set of good habits. There are simple versions of these techniques that people may use on their own, but they are most effective when working with a psychotherapist. Studies on large groups of people find that combining the two techniques is most effective; however, some individuals are helped more by one or the other. Cognitive-behavioral strategies are helpful when people cling to excuses discussed in earlier chapters: that they're genetically incapable of losing weight or that they're always going to start that exercise regime tomorrow. Hypnosis and other imagery techniques work especially well for people with vivid imaginations. They can learn to block hunger or impulses in much the same way that hypnosis can block even strong pain signals. They can experience success in their imagery—enjoying low-calorie foods, developing athletic skill and achieving their ideal weight—before they have to make the change. This can be enormously motivating. I'll describe how both techniques work and give examples from patients in my practice.

Cognitive-Behavioral Therapy. This approach has its roots in the work of George Kelly, described above, and that of Albert Ellis, who focused on irrational thoughts as the basis of his clients' emotional problems. Ellis sang ditties about those irrationalities in an off-key nasal twang and preached against "musturbation," defined as the destructive idea that our needs and expectations must be met. Cognitive-behavioral therapy proper began with Aaron Beck, who shared the idea that faulty beliefs caused difficulties but who was less flamboyant than either Kelly or Ellis.

Cognitive-behavioral therapists ask clients to keep a log of occurrences of the problem—for excess weight, simply charting everything one eats and any exercise. Recording eating makes it less automatic and sometimes this alone decreases intake or encourages healthier choices. Clients are also asked to note *when* they overeat, what external cues were present—and most importantly, what their thoughts were. These automatic thoughts are then examined for faulty reasoning and possible alternate ways of construing the situation. Some faulty thinking becomes transparent to the client just by writing it down—if, for instance, every time someone goes to get coffee at a donut shop, they end up with at least one donut, or if reasoning that they can eat a large lunch as long as they eat a small supper never actually results in the latter. Other self-defeating thoughts are not as obvious until the therapist questions them, and one must work on finding alternatives. Here are a few of the most common patterns:

"It's genetic," "I'm built that way," "I don't eat much; I just can't lose weight." Most people who think they're eating very little are underestimating calories, and forgetting, and fudging. A research tool called "doubly labeled water" can medically measure how many calories a person has consumed. When this is compared with dieters' self-reports, studies find that over-weight people report 81 percent of their actual consumption and obese people report 64 percent—a few obese individuals report less than 50 percent of what they've actually eaten.[13] So it's helpful to train people in accurate caloric estimation.

Some people believe there's no diet on which they would lose weight. But if you ask if there's an intake—even zero—at which they'd starve, they definitely think they could starve to death. That helps set up a framework—"At halfway between your present intake and zero, what do you think would happen?"—from which they can estimate how many calories they should be consuming. Of course it may be genetic that one has to eat less than others to stay at a healthy weight, but, as we've seen with the Pima research, there's no such thing as genes that don't interact with diet and exercise. A closely related belief is that one can't lose weight because "this is the way I always ate" or "these are the foods I grew up with." But just as with genetics, it's not impossible for people who grew up with poor eating habits to change, it's just harder. Which brings us to the next category.

"It's not fair." "Other people pig out and aren't even overweight." Life isn't fair. We all basically know that, but we can hang onto a childlike insistence otherwise when we're holding the short end of the stick. Ellis would sing his goofy, plaintive "Life really owes me the things that I miss, Fate has to grant me eternal bliss. . . ." But often the best way to reframe this is a variation on "count your blessings." Yes, a client may be unfortunate in metabolism, but most people can easily name some way in which they've won life's lotteries: great kids, great spouse, interesting job, good friends. Even the few who don't count personal blessings can name somewhere else on the planet (usually most of it) where they're glad they weren't born. Thinking about the ways in which one is fortunate can make it more bearable to have to work harder in one particular area than others do.

"I need to have dessert and snacks around in case company drops by." "My husband isn't on a diet, so I still need to buy potato chips for him." "Little Johnny loves ice cream; I have to have that in the house." Sometimes, when you inquire further, it turns out that company never actually drops by. If they do, they're never dropping by to see what's to eat. In fact, the client says they often demur: "Oh dear, no, I'm trying to lose weight." Thin family members will benefit almost as much from eating healthier foods—albeit perhaps larger servings—as the dieter. I often tell clients about a Dutch study showing that the number of years lost from life is higher for eating unhealthy food than for being overweight per se.[14] Of course little Johnny loves ice cream; he'd love cigarettes by now if his parents had been been doling those out after dinner. Again, unhealthy eating is slightly deadlier than cigarettes.[15] It's often even the same people who blame their weight problem on what their parents fed them who also mention needing to have junk food in the house for their kids. Usually a therapist can persuade clients that they don't need to keep separate, unhealthy foods for guests or family—and can enlist others in changing their eating habits simultaneously. If not, it's necessary to brainstorm whether to segregate—or even hide—these other foods, or whether to begin to practice Rankin's willpower techniques.

Most thoughts have an easy substitute: "I've got too much to lose—I could never shed all these pounds." That doesn't make it impossible, it just means it takes longer; it translates into "So it's more important to start now." Other clients say, "I need to reward/comfort myself after a rough day." It's not a reward to take years off your life, diminish your energy and intellectual capacity, depress yourself and increase the odds of painful diseases. These are things we shouldn't wish on our worst enemies. A healthy reward is massage, yoga, a DVD of your favorite concerto/punk rock, a call to a friend you've been wanting to catch up with. Plus, just feeling good about how you are taking care of your body, the way you would feel proud of caring well for a child or a pet, can be reinforcing in itself—clients need to begin to label the healthy, light meal or the run as a reward. Clients chart such new self-talk, first in the service of making it more conscious, and eventually making it a habit.

Hypnosis. Most studies of hypnosis for weight loss find that patients lose weight. The amount of weight loss varies, mostly with the length of the treatment period.[16] In one study, after eight weeks of sessions with a hypnotist and twelve weeks of practicing self-hypnosis, subjects lost an average of twenty pounds.[17] Another compared group hypnosis with individualized procedures and found that both led to weight loss but those using an individualized approach lost more.[18] Hypnosis has also been found to increase compliance with an exercise program even in patients who weren't trying to lose weight.[19]

Research indicates that adding hypnosis to a cognitive-behavioral weight management program results in more weight loss than the cognitive-behavioral treatment alone.[20] A meta-analysis, or combined re-analysis of many of these studies of varying lengths, found that the benefits of hypnosis increased over time. Averaged over different periods of measurement, there was a weight loss of six pounds without hypnosis and almost twelve pounds with hypnosis. At the last assessment period, the gap was still widening, with the same loss of six pounds without but fifteen pounds with hypnosis.[21]

People vary greatly in their hypnotizability. Although the myth is that "weak-willed" or gullible people are more hypnotizable, the traits that actually predict response to hypnosis are vividness of imagination, ability to block out real physical stimuli and a history of entering spontaneous trancelike states. If you had imaginary playmates as a child, can vividly picture a person or place not actually in front of you and take more than usual calling to get your attention if you're engrossed in a book, you're likelier to be hypnotizable. People who live exclusively in their immediate physical environment, don't fantasize and don't know how to tune out distracting stimuli except by physically escaping from them are likely to be less hypnotizable.[22] Several studies confirm the general clinical impression that people of higher hypnotizability benefit most from hypnotherapy for weight loss.[23]

Suggestions given for weight loss during hypnosis include some combination of telling clients they will enjoy low-calorie, healthy foods and feel satisfied after small servings. It's suggested that they won't crave problem foods—that these begin to look nasty, toxic or unreal, or that they just lose interest in them. Phrasing that I often use is *"finding to your surprise* that you" just ignore rich foods or go the whole time between meals without thinking about eating. People of high hypnotizability will often repeat back to me in the next session something like, "To my surprise, I went all afternoon without even thinking about food," seemingly unaware that this was in their instructions.

Hypnosis also gives people a sneak preview of what achieving their goals will be like. They can vividly experience stepping on scales and seeing a lower number, noticing that clothes zip easier, or their long-term goals: being slim again, having energy for sports, a physician giving them a good health report, knowing they're going to be there to see their grandchild grow up. For high-hypnotizables, these visions of the future are dramatic. And for them, suggestions can make them *really not feel hunger or cravings*. This is not actually so surprising—hunger may be as powerful as pain, but not more so. These are the same people who would get complete pain relief with hypnosis as the only anesthesia. Pain and hunger are both survival signals, but they can both be overridden in people of high hypnotizability, so hypnotherapists are careful not to suggest that a client will never be hungry at all.

For people of moderate hypnotizability, imagery of a positive outcome motivates them even though it doesn't have the same hallucinatory quality. The hypnotist's verbal phrases come to mind at times of temptation to reinforce their goals— they just don't get the same complete free pass on physical cravings as their bodies adjust to the changes. To give readers a better feel for what goes on in hypnosis for weight loss, the following is a summary of my recent work with one young woman of moderate hypnotizability.

Toni was a twenty-five-year-old who came to hypnotherapy for weight loss. As I questioned her about the history of her weight, it was a typical story. She'd been not exactly thin, but not heavy through high school. She ran on the track team. At college, she gained what today's undergrads refer to as the "freshman fifteen"—and then sophomore and junior pounds too. Her running became occasional Sunday recreation and the distance dropped.

After graduation, Toni took a sedentary computer-programming job. The running stopped entirely. Her coworkers were men who lived on delivered pepperoni pizzas and little donuts from the snack machines. They didn't seem to care about their own appearance and she didn't care what they thought of hers. She began to dress like them, in baggy jeans and T-shirts.

In addition to wanting to get back to athletics, and just not to huff too badly on the stairs when the elevator was broken, Toni's other motive for losing weight was to "look good in anime costumes." *Anime?* I vaguely knew the term: animation films out of Japan for teens and young adults, human and humanoid characters, heavy on sci-fi content. I didn't know they generated conventions—much like those of *Star Trek* fans—regional, national and international. The best were in Japan.

"I have to be an animal character or some funny sidekick, not the femme fatale," Toni lamented. "There are all these sexy women, like Battle Angel Alita who wears a silver metallic bodysuit, that I can't possibly be."

Toni was of at least average hypnotizability, so when I talked her through one of the runs she used to love, she saw the river, the dogwood buds, felt the impact of her sneakers on the damp path and experienced the rush she used to get running. I told her this old part of herself would return and she'd find herself automatically yearning to go out for a run again.

I described the salads and broiled chicken and fruit she'd enjoy eating again. Told her how revolting the cold puddles of grease on the pizzas would look. That she'd find herself ignoring the snack machine, and perceive the little packets her coworkers extracted from it as resembling damp foam rubber. I described—fed back, really—the description she'd given me of her android's silver lamé catsuit, so that she would see herself as the perfect embodiment of the character.

Toni began to run again. She brought salad to work and

eschewed the snack machines, passed on pizza with the guys. She lost thirty pounds before the next anime convention. She went as Super Cat Girl Nuku Nuku—bosomy, hardly thin but no longer a comical character. She returned, ran, began to take anime magazines to work to entertain herself while the guys were snacking. Lost another twenty-five pounds. Went to the next meeting as almost thin Vampire Princess Miyu. The silver-laméd Battle Angel Alita was in sight.

What We Can Learn from Anorexics

This is one group of people who actually *are* too thin. Obviously, I'm not advocating a delusional body image or starving oneself. Anorexia nervosa is a serious disorder that can kill. But it has an interesting relationship to obesity. The current, politically correct interpretation is that anorexia is on the rise because of our culture's over-concern with weight and its "unrealistically thin ideal." However, there were always thin people around and they were often idealized, as discussed in Chapter 6. What's different now is the number of *obese* people and the genuinely high risk of becoming overweight by young adulthood. It's hard to become afraid of being fat without seeing lots of fat people, or have a distorted image of one's body as terribly obese without having seen such bodies.

But the most interesting aspect of anorexia for our purposes is that *these are people who know how to take weight off.* They're succeeding in their diet goals—however misguided—while most of America is failing. In working with anorexics on inpatient psychiatric wards, I've been struck by the power of their techniques. They know that the first couple of days of calorie restriction are by far the hardest and that sudden intense hunger usually passes within thirty minutes even without eating. They sound much like fasting religious mystics when they describe how one can

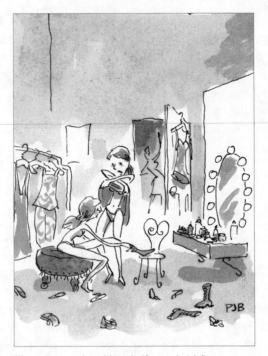

"I'm so hungry I could eat half a sandwich."
(© *The New Yorker Collection 1998 Pat Byrnes*
from cartoonbank.com)

learn to experience hunger as pleasurable. They know what athletes do about pushing past the first resistance to exercise and entering the "runners' high." They are experts at fending off people trying to sabotage their diet. Of course, anorexics display an excess of these strategies, but most dieters display a deficit. Some of the way my thinking changed while working with these people is illustrated in the following clinical vignette.

Todd had regained fifteen pounds. With an anorexic's distinctive dual thinking, he could acknowledge that 110 pounds for a 6'4" man was dangerously thin; still he looked fat to himself. I'd tried every standard cognitive reality-testing strategy I could think of, to no avail. Then, unexpectedly, he talked with the only other anorexic on unit—Sarah, five years older and a veteran of many hospitalizations. Sarah told Todd that as he regained weight, it first went to his stomach and made that fat, but that if he just endured this for a few weeks and exercised hard, gradually the new weight would redistribute to arms, legs and chest as muscle.

Todd was so relieved by this, he told me he could now let himself gain more weight. I was thankful for anything that had this effect and stored it away as something to tell other anorexics in the future. I repeatedly did, always to good effect. But at this point I thought of it as a weird misperception that anorexics shared—not quite true but true to their perception. At most, I thought that food in their stomachs made that area slightly heavier relative to their emaciated bodies. But later I began to see their midsections unclothed and realized it was actually true. It's not just food in the stomach, but two or three pounds of glycogen in the liver, and pounds of fat cells in the abdomen. Just like starving African children with distended stomachs, anorexics can have a pot belly and still be starving.

At the time, my supervisors viewed exercise as almost as bad as self-starvation, but Sarah was right on this point, too. Young adults practically can't exercise too hard unless their muscles have atrophied. Exercise will direct calories away from abdominal fat toward muscle. I now encourage exercise for anorexics except for the few with cardiac conditions.

I know many stories of anorexics who've gotten together and taught each other their worst tricks: how to eat fiber, which digests slowest, ahead of simple starches that would otherwise pass through the stomach quickly so that the stomach doesn't empty and they can vomit up to one and a half hours after a meal when staff has quit observing them; how to use the occupational therapy clay to sculpt a couple of pounds around their genitals that won't be detected during their underwear-clad weigh-ins. But this time Todd learned something useful—and so did I.

As anorexics recover and realize they're emaciated, not obese, their control over what they eat often serves them well in establishing new healthy diets. Many adopt regimens that echo their previous obsessiveness, but with healthy specifics. They usually continue to get a lot of exercise. Some recovered anorexics have lingering physical problems—most commonly acidic tooth decay if they induced vomiting frequently. However, several studies have found that people with a history of anorexia have a significantly lower incidence of cancer years and decades later.[24] The most common interpretation is that the anorexic period lowered their exposure to estrogen, insulin-like growth factor and other hormones that stimulate cancer. I suspect that not just the anorexic's history but the rigidity with which some of them continue to eat at their new, acceptable weight has something to do with this. One thing anorexia demonstrates is that rigid diets are not inherently harder to follow than looser ones.

What We Can Learn from Religious Diets

As mentioned in Chapter 7, the few religious denominations that still discourage gluttony are slimmer than others, as are the Amish who insist on vigorous manual labor. More common in religious diets are prohibitions against specific foods or drinks. Muslims and kosher Jews don't eat pork; Mormons don't drink anything containing caffeine; Muslims and some fundamentalist Christian denominations prohibit alcohol. Even though these rules aren't going to make people much slimmer or fitter, what's relevant is that these are substances most people would find it hard to forgo; indeed, many fail when they try to limit these same substances for other reasons. For the religious, however, it's a willing sacrifice; they can follow these diets their whole lives with satisfaction. Granted, the rules are begrudged and cheated on by coerced offspring or half-hearted believers. But true believers are so committed to avoiding forbidden food and drink that they don't even think about it—it's a habit. The same is true for physical exertion. Hundreds of thousands of Tibetan Buddhists make the pilgrimage to the holy Mount Kailash on foot from as much as three thousand miles away—a few bowing every step of the way. They find great satisfaction in the effort. Compare that to what secular folks find too demanding by way of exercise.

Some religious followers have broad social support for their practices. Mormons in Salt Lake City, Jews within an orthodox neighborhood or Muslims in a country with Islamic laws have the easiest time following their religion's diet. In the next chapter, I'll discuss how we might structure our society to make healthy eating and exercise this automatic. But the fact that a family, a few friends or a lone individual can follow religious prescriptions in a society that indulges in alcohol, caffeine and pork—this has an important message for those of us who don't want to wait for our society to change. Religious diets succeed largely by having very absolute, clear rules, taking seriously how important those rules are and following them consistently so that they become habits.

Successful Losers

The National Weight Control Registry[25] was founded in 1993 to study the characteristics of people who successfully maintained weight loss for at least a year. People sign up online and give self-reported data via an electronic questionnaire. The accuracy of this data is not ideally rigorous, but it is by far the largest study of successful weight loss—the registry includes more than

4,500 individuals. The average registrant reports a loss of sixty pounds maintained for five years. About half of the participants lost weight entirely on their own. About half had some kind of nutritional or behavioral counseling in an individual or group setting—these were spread across a wide variety of approaches.

The vast majority of the registry members follow rigorous diet and exercise regimes for maintenance. On average, they report eating 1,380 calories per day. That number is at least as low as the much thinner CR Society members, and it may be that the registry people underestimate their calories as much as the 20 percent average for dieters in other studies. Although their initial weight-loss diets varied greatly, including some low-carb high-fat diets, once they had successfully lost the weight they tended to eat low-fat as well as low-calorie diets, with an average 24 percent of their calories from fat. They report very high levels of physical activity—enough to burn about 2,800 calories a week. The standard "expert" advice to people who want to lose weight is to expend 1,000 calories a week. Burning 2,800 calories is equivalent to walking twenty-eight miles a week, or about three to four miles a day. However, these people get less than half their exercise walking and additionally many are bicycling, taking aerobics classes and using stair-climbing machines. A fair number do high-intensity activities like step aerobics, weightlifting and running.

Diet "experts" usually discourage frequent weighing on the basis of unproven rationales; however, half of the registry members weigh themselves every day and 75 percent weigh themselves at least once a week. They tended to say it was important to keep close tabs on the first sign of any increase. And, though conventional wisdom also holds that it's harder to maintain than to lose weight, registry members don't say that. Half of them report that maintaining weight is actually easier than losing it; most of the rest judge the tasks equal.

Two-thirds of these successful weight losers were overweight as children. Sixty percent report a family history of obesity—radically challenging the notion that genetics is a major factor in who can lose weight. Encouragingly for other Americans, most of the registrants had one or more failed diet attempts before hitting on their successful regimen. Most of these previous attempts were less rigorous; sometimes the registrants said they were simply less motivated on their previous attempts. Ninety-five percent said that the overall quality of their lives had improved, and 92 percent said that their level of energy was greater since their weight loss.[26]

The registry members demonstrate most of the same principles as religious groups and the CR Society. It is possible to pick a rigorous diet and exercise program and adhere to it consistently. But for an overwhelming majority this is not happening—despite the risks of painful chronic illness and earlier death. It's obviously desirable to change the environment into one that supports healthy habits instead of one that encourages overeating and immobility. The next chapter will explore this alternative.

9

Changing the Drumbeat:
Strategies for a
Healthy Society

If we want to make our community, or country, or world slimmer and fitter, the solution lies beyond individual strategies for resisting our supernormal environment. It means changing the world we live in, not just how we live in it. Education and political action are needed to change food and exercise options back to something compatible with our genetic programming.

In many ways, the prospects for change look bleak. Our government subsidizes the production of unhealthy foods instead of wholesome ones; each year, more farm products go into refined, packaged junk food. Tens of thousands of fast-food outlets open each year—we're up to 500,000 in the US alone—many of them financed by government start-up grants. In 2005, Americans spent $100 billion on fast food, more than on higher education, personal computers, software or new cars. We're gaining weight so rapidly that epidemiologists project that by 2020, two-thirds rather than the present one-third of Americans will be obese. The National Institutes of Health estimates that the average lifespan of Americans will drop by five years because of

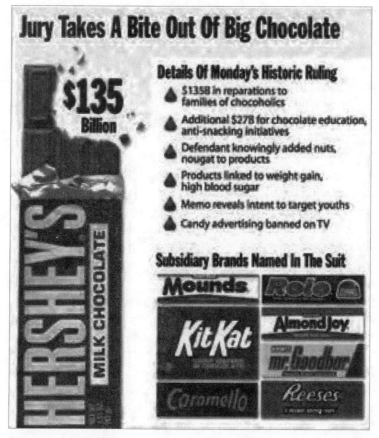

Jury Takes A Bite Out Of Big Chocolate

$135 Billion

Details Of Monday's Historic Ruling

▲ $135B in reparations to families of chocoholics

▲ Additional $27B for chocolate education, anti-snacking initiatives

▲ Defendant knowingly added nuts, nougat to products

▲ Products linked to weight gain, high blood sugar

▲ Memo reveals intent to target youths

▲ Candy advertising banned on TV

Subsidiary Brands Named In The Suit

Mounds Rolo KitKat Almond Joy mr. Goodbar Caramello Reeses

HERSHEY'S MILK CHOCOLATE

(Courtesy of The Onion)

rising obesity. America is the fattest of any major country, but the rest of the world is close behind.

The good news is that the US once led the world in rates of smoking and lung cancer deaths but, for the last two decades, it finally leads the world in smoking cessation, anti-tobacco legislation and declines in lung cancer. The first signs of a similar mobilization against junk food and physical inactivity are already evident. As described in Chapter 3, a new agreement by vendors reduces the number of sugary and high-fat offerings in school snack machines. Some states have instituted adult exercise programs. One recent lawsuit charged McDonald's with causing two girls' obesity and a second accused several chains of causing a 270-pound Bronx maintenance worker's heart attack.

The lawsuits were widely ridiculed before being dismissed as frivolous. However, "That's what they said about the smoking lawsuits," says John Banzhaf. A law professor at George Washington University, Banzhaf was among the first to sue tobacco companies and now the food chains. "The fast-food industry does not regard these suits as ludicrous or frivolous. They've hired a PR firm to run attack ads, they write op-ed pieces, and according to a trade publication the National Restaurant Association has gone to Congress seeking protection from the suits, and they are actively trying out health warnings of the kind they ought to be providing."[1]

As this book goes to press, the US House of Representatives has passed Bill 554, nicknamed the Cheeseburger Bill. This bill is promoted by the food industry and, if the Senate passes the virtually identical Bill 908, it will become more difficult to sue food companies for the health effects of their products.[2] Also passed by the House and now before the Senate is a bill which would prohibit states from requiring stricter health warnings on foods than those legislated by the federal government.[3] These bills, if passed, would present temporary setbacks to health initiatives, but their very existence demonstrates, as Banzhaf argues, that food companies are very worried about their long-term prospects for business as usual.

In the 1970s, suggesting limits on even where someone could smoke was viewed as an infringement on basic rights. The anti-smoking campaign can be an excellent model for obesity action: education shifting to emphatic warning labels for adults, outright prohibition of sales to children and financial incentives to grow and sell healthy food in reasonable portions. One powerful government institution already holds the power to regulate some of these aspects of our food.

The Fox in Charge of the Henhouse

The United States Department of Agriculture sets most of our country's official nutritional policy. Many Americans assume that the USDA exists, at least in part, to enhance our good health. But that is not its mission. The department was established to promote agricultural products. Most of us want to see the American farmer succeed, but even this isn't the USDA's main interest. Its boards are loaded with food-company executives. Its policies favor big agriculture and refined-food producers. In the words of former Senator Peter Fitzgerald, a veteran of the Senate Agricultural Committee, "Putting the USDA in charge of dietary advice is in some respects like putting the fox in charge of the henhouse."[4] Let's look in more detail at the USDA's major functions before discussing how these should change.

Subsidies. The USDA doles out $19 billion annually in subsidies to farmers. Small amounts of this money occasionally go to vegetables or fruit, but the vast majority goes toward such unhealthy foods as white flour, white rice, butter and oils to be turned into hydrogenated margarine. In the years 2000–02, the USDA provided $299 million to subsidize the production of corn, much of which is turned directly into corn syrup. During the same period, the USDA paid $479 million to tobacco farmers while putting not a dime toward incentives to grow broccoli, spinach, farmed salmon—or any food proven healthy by medical research.[5] Lest one think subsidies exist to prevent shortages, it's the opposite. Agricultural subsidies were introduced in the 1920s as a reaction to crop surpluses which drove down prices. As a post–World War I emergency measure, this may have made sense, but it has become an entrenched part of the

American economy that is also hampering international trade agreements, since foreign farmers understandably view US farm subsidies as unfair competition. Attempts to do away with subsidies have met with crushing resistance. The 1996 Freedom to Farm Act was passed supposedly to end them, but they were replaced with barely distinguishable fixed payments and "emergency payments" to farmers for virtually the same crops. By 2000 crop subsidies had tripled from the 1996 level.[6]

Grading. The USDA's Agricultural Marketing Service spends about $297 million a year on functions such as grading commodities to help market them. In its "Fact Sheet on Inspection and Grading of Beef," the USDA describes its grades:

- "Prime" meat has the highest marbling with fat
- "Choice" has a high but slightly lesser percent fat
- "Select" has a bit less fat yet
- "Regular" cuts of meat have the least fat

When cancer, heart disease and an early death are all correlated with the amount of saturated fat eaten, does it make any sense to label the fattiest meat "Prime"? Well, yes, to be fair—by one criterion it does. Our taste buds and cravings tell us it is. Centuries of breeding cattle for excess fat have produced the perfect supernormal stimulus. Even "Regular" cuts of meat are fattier than the wild game of our hunter-gatherer ancestors. High-fat tastes best to us. However, when our government uses taxpayers' money to direct us toward what to eat, should hedonistic craving be reinforced? Or would we perhaps prefer a grading system that reinforced the decisions of our evolved brain about what's wisest to eat?

Parenthetically, the same fact sheet also volunteers, "The dye used to stamp the grade and inspection marks onto a meat carcass is made from a food-grade vegetable dye and is not harmful."[7] Why do they feel the need to assure us that their current dye is not harmful? Because the previous dye for stamping

"Prime" on the fattiest cuts of meat, Violet Dye No. 1, was banned after research showed that it was a carcinogen.[8]

US Dietary Guidelines, Including the Food Pyramid. The nation's dietary guidelines and the food guide pyramid are crafted by the USDA's Center for Nutrition Policy and Promotion and revised every five years. Eric Hentges, director of the center, spent over fifteen years working for the meat industry, most recently the National Pork Board. Other committee members have ties to Campbell's Soup, Procter & Gamble, the American Cocoa Research Institute, the Sugar Association, the Kellogg Company and the Wisconsin Milk Marketing Board.[9] The USDA provides Hentges with twenty-eight employees and $2.8 million a year to run its nutrition programs.

It used to be that the guidelines were solely the work of this center; more recently, the Department of Health and Human Services has been enlisted for advice. Ahead of the most recent revision of the guidelines, Senator Fitzgerald—the USDA's most outspoken critic—introduced a bill that would have moved them entirely to HHS. He suggested that this department would "start out with an orientation toward science and less coziness with the farm groups." After vigorous lobbying against it by the food industry, this proposal failed.

The revision presented the chance to reword recommendations that nutritionists judged to be too vague in the previous guidelines such as:

- about fats: "Choose a diet that is low in saturated fat and cholesterol and moderate in total fat," and
- about carbohydrates: "Choose beverages and foods to moderate your intake of sugars."

Twenty-five nutrition professors across the country signed a joint letter urging the USDA to clearly lay out what people should and should not eat with specific wording:

- about fats: "Eat less cheese, beef, pork, whole and 2% milk, egg yolks, pastries and other foods that are high in saturated fat, trans-fat or cholesterol," and
- about carbohydrates: "Drink fewer soft drinks and limit cake, cookies, frozen desserts and other foods rich in refined sugars."

What did the committee do? They ignored this advice and further watered down the old wording to omit any hint of discouragement of specific foods such as sugar. The new guidelines' equivalent sentences are ludicrously vague:

- about fats: "Choose fats wisely for good health," and
- about carbohydrates: "Choose carbohydrates wisely."

Fitzgerald also encouraged the committee to dramatically revise the food pyramid. He believes the pyramid reflects the department's close ties with grain and sugar producers. Waving a box of crackers in a hearing on the topic, Fitzgerald pointed out that it displayed the food guide pyramid and touted the crackers as part of the USDA's recommended six to eleven daily servings of grain. Yet the label showed that five crackers contained more carbohydrates than two Krispy Kreme doughnuts. "The pyramid is giving a government stamp of approval to these products," he complained. "I think the guidelines are fundamentally flawed and misleading."

Other aspects of the food pyramid are equally vague. "The dairy group mixes fat-free milk with high-fat cheese," Fitzgerald observed. "The protein group mixes fatty meats with wholesome beans." Even though his attempts at reform failed, it was the first time that the shortcomings in the pyramid had been so well publicized. Fitzgerald's flamboyant advocacy may have set the stage for reform next time around. The Department of Agriculture's current program, he said, "probably has more to do with diabetes and obesity than Krispy Kremes."

Marketing. The USDA's Agricultural Marketing Services also oversee "checkoff" programs that require producers to set aside a percentage of each sale, which a USDA board then uses for generic promotions and advertising. The beef checkoff receives $80 million a year for promotion. It has used the money to coin the slogan, "Beef: it's what's for dinner" and provide funding for a touring Beefmobile. The program provided its logo and endorsement to Domino's Pizza for its Philly Cheese Steak Pizza.

The pork checkoff, meanwhile, collects $60 million a year for such projects as drafting the slogan "The other white meat." The dairy and milk promotion programs, with a budget of $200 million, fund the milk mustache ad campaign ("Got milk?") and coax fast-food chains to develop cheesier pizzas, quesadillas and cheeseburgers, including Wendy's Cheddar Lovers' Bacon Cheeseburger. The Dairy Board "assisted Wendy's with the development of this cheese-friendly sandwich," according to the board's 1999 annual report. When Pizza Hut unveiled its "Summer of Cheese" campaign it featured two recipes developed with help from the board: the Stuffed Crust Pizza and the Insider. "We helped Pizza Hut develop those pizzas, so we made sure they use a lot of cheese," the board's then chairman, Paul Rovey, said. "Look what happened: the 'Summer of Cheese' at Pizza Hut moved 100 million pounds of cheese."[10]

USDA officials say the checkoff programs are funded entirely by industry, but nutrition professor Marion Nestle describes them as "federally sanctioned and administered public relations enterprises to benefit certain food commodities." Food growers who don't want to participate have challenged checkoffs in court, arguing that they violate free speech and force small producers to contribute to advertising that favors their larger competitors. Courts have preliminarily agreed that the programs are unconstitutional, but those rulings have been appealed. The programs continue to promote cheesier cheeseburgers and cheese steak pizza until the appeal process is complete. And the legal action hasn't even addressed the unhealthiness of the promotions, only the unfairness of making small producers finance them.

Getting Chickens and Eggs Away from the Fox

Of all these functions, subsidies to farmers and food grading are the only two that properly belong with the USDA. These need a major overhaul dictated by Congress to revise what we want to subsidize. Corn syrup, butter and margarine are obviously out. Grains and milk products are healthy enough in modest amounts of their optimum versions—whole grains, non-fat milk and cheese—but they don't need subsidies to keep these more modest quantities in existence. Dark green leafy vegetables, tomatoes, berries, fish farmed with feed low in mercury and PCBs—these are the types of agricultural products we want to subsidize in the future. Farmers would be harmed if we cut subsidies—and some will resist any change. But they're not out to kill us; most would get behind a switch as long as they were paid at least as well. And while we're at it, tobacco farmers should be transitioned over to growing non-lethal crops.

Likewise, any mandatory product promotion should be for healthy food. Soy is one of the few healthy crops that already receive subsidies—and this on top of having a great market as animal feed. However, it could use some help with its consumer image as a human food. Slogans for soy. Slogans for fish. Slogans for broccoli instead of presidents who announce their distaste for it. We want the next think tank sitting around debating whether it violates separation of church and state if their check-off slogan read "What did Jesus feed the throngs?" over a picture

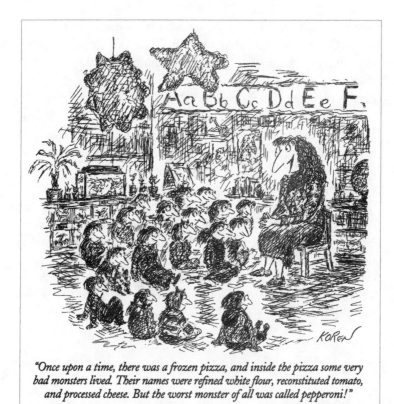

"*Once upon a time, there was a frozen pizza, and inside the pizza some very bad monsters lived. Their names were refined white flour, reconstituted tomato, and processed cheese. But the worst monster of all was called pepperoni!*"

(© The New Yorker Collection 2000 Edward Koren from cartoonbank.com)

of multiplying fish and whole wheat loaves. (Er, yes, it *does* violate it.)

For other health policies such as the nutritional guidelines, the USDA just isn't the right branch of government. As Senator Fitzgerald observed, "I see a lot of cozy relationships every day in Washington that probably work out to the detriment of taxpayers. But in this case, the coziness is more troubling. We are talking about their health and their lives."[11] He's hardly alone in this observation. "The USDA clearly has a conflict of interest," said Michael Jacobson, executive director of the Center for Science in the Public Interest. "The USDA doesn't want to offend any sector of the agriculture industry. Nutrition advocates should be encouraging people to eat less meat, to eat less cheese and sugar. It's tough for the USDA to say those things."[12]

The proper department for nutritional advice is indeed Health and Human Services. By the next time the guidelines are revised in 2010, we should see that the job is delegated to that department. The appropriate people to sit on the revision committee are not those with ties to food companies. The twenty-five nutrition professors who wrote the letter which the last committee ignored include such luminaries as Marion Nestle of NYU—several of them would be a good start. And medical researchers like Walter Willett, Stanley B. Eaton and Luigi Fontana, whom I quoted in Chapters 2 and 7 about research on which foods result in the longest life and least illness—these are the people we want telling us what to eat.

The FDA versus Vitamins

Another branch of the government that needs to change its input into our nutrition is the Food and Drug Administration. Their philosophy has been that people should be able to get all vitamins and other nutrients from food and therefore supplements are unnecessary for routine health. However, a large government study recently found that the average American is not getting enough vitamin E, vitamin A, vitamin C or magnesium—in fact, 93 percent of Americans have a deficiency of vitamin E.[13] Other studies have found that between 42 and 57 percent of Americans are deficient in vitamin D.[14]

Even in light of these data, the FDA opposes supplements, arguing that taking vitamins causes people to neglect to eat healthy food. The opposite relationship has been demonstrated in study after study, however; people who take vitamins and other supplements are the same ones who eat healthy food. People who don't take supplements are also the ones getting the fewest vitamins from food. And even though we wish the FDA's confidence in the vitamin content of food was well-founded, with all the selective breeding research we know this is not necessarily assured.

Until recently, the FDA spent much of its attention to supplements in censoring health claims that it deemed unsubstantiated. Most of these were not wild, fraudulent claims but ones tied to the findings of mainstream research studies. A supplement manufacturer finally challenged this process in federal court when the FDA banned four of its product statements that had considerable scientific evidence:

- Consumption of antioxidant vitamins may reduce the risk of certain kinds of cancers.
- Consumption of fiber may reduce the risk of colorectal cancer.
- Consumption of omega-3 fatty acids may reduce the risk of coronary heart disease.
- 800 mcg of folic acid in a dietary supplement is more effective in reducing the risk of neural tube defects than a lower amount in foods.

The court held that the FDA's health claims review standards were so vague as to be unconstitutional. It ordered the FDA to implement new, clear standards (it has yet to do this) and mandated that it allow the four claims even if they failed to satisfy that new review standard. The court ruled that the only constitutional right the FDA has on the issue of health claims is to insist on reasonably worded disclaimers such as "These statements have not been evaluated by the Food and Drug Administration."

Even with its banning power curtailed, the FDA still seems to be spending much of its nutrition money lobbying against vitamins. It would be better if it allowed—or even actively endorsed—the idea that a multivitamin and mineral supplement is beneficial for maintaining optimal health.

Eliminating Corporate Welfare in Favor of the General Welfare

"For Big Franchises, Money to Go: Is the SBA Dispensing Corporate Welfare?" asked a 1997 *Washington Post* article. The answer is yes. Small Business Administration (SBA) loans are another example of the government structuring incentives in the wrong direction. The loans were established to help entrepreneurs start small businesses, but they've evolved into something which helps corporations put independents out of business. The loophole is that SBA loans can be used to open a franchise of a national corporation—including fast-food chains. Most of the loan start-up money goes to the corporation; the small business owner is paying a hefty franchise fee on top of construction of the outlet, its dictated furnishings, kitchen equipment and suppliers. If the outlet fails, the corporation has no investment to lose—but the taxpayer does. Between 1967 and 1979, eighteen thousand franchise loans were granted, many to fast-food outlets. The loan recipients defaulted on loans at a rate of 10 percent—far more than for non-franchise loans.[15]

In 1996 alone, the SBA granted $1 billion in franchise loans. Most critics want simply to redirect this money to independent businesses where start-up costs go to local construction companies and a variety of suppliers. But there's another direction in which to revamp this program: a requirement could be instituted that the new businesses serve a beneficial purpose—or at least that they do no harm. A proposal for a restaurant or store that would sell primarily high-fiber, high-vitamin whole foods would be eligible for a loan. A restaurant to sell cheeseburgers or ice cream wouldn't—nor would someone proposing yet another "convenience store" selling donuts, potato chips and cigarettes. It's far short of banning them not to help finance them.

Taxation is another route to non-compulsory incentives. States have standard sales tax rates for most goods with food taxed not at all, lower than or equal to the standard sales tax. In all states, cigarettes and alcohol are taxed at higher rates than other commodities. This is simultaneously an attempt to reduce consumption (research indicates price does make a difference) and to provide funds to ameliorate damage caused by these products. Most of Europe taxes gasoline at similarly high rates to encourage fuel-efficient cars, keep pollution down and conserve fossil fuel supplies. A similar strategy could work with unhealthy foods. If foods in which saturated fats and refined sugar or flour make up the majority of calories were taxed at several times the rate of apples, tomatoes and fish, it wouldn't end junk food consumption, but it would reduce it.

Many people object to such proposals as paternalistic. Those who eat low-nutrition sweets and snacks only occasionally see it as unnecessary—but it's hardly going to make a noticeable difference in their grocery tabs. People who end up paying hefty amounts in such tax will get this back at the other end in health and disability payments, which we're now hard-pressed to provide for in our growing diet-related health crisis. When we buy wine for our homes or order the occasional glass in a restaurant, we generally accept that we're paying a liquor tax higher than we pay on food. It seems natural that we pay more for such non-necessities. The only difference in this versus a proposed junk-food tax is that the one on alcohol has been in existence long enough for us to get used to it.

Labeling the most egregious offenders with health warnings is another method by which dietary initiatives can emulate efforts against tobacco. No one was getting the information for the first time in 1964 when their cigarette packs began to state that the Surgeon General had determined that smoking causes cancer and birth defects. But over the years, these warnings gradually discouraged smokers. Similarly, few are unaware of the links between sugar and overeating and diabetes, but it might improve eating habits to label some foods: "Eating refined sugar and flour will increase your chances of diabetes, which can result in kidney failure, blindness and amputations." On others: "Saturated fats increase the risk of cancer and heart attack," or "Eating more than the recommended daily calories increases your chances of early death and Alzheimer's disease." This may sound extreme, but I can remember the days when cigarette companies had people convinced that similar statements about

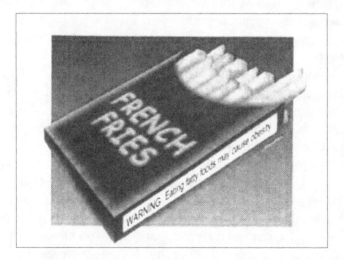

(Courtesy of The Onion*)*

cigarettes were radical and were still describing well-established adverse health effects of tobacco as "unproven."

Advertising regulation is another way to reduce junk-food consumption without totally forbidding specific products. In 2004, Congress asked the Centers for Disease Control and Prevention to examine the effects of advertising foods directly to children. Their book-length response details 123 scientific studies which establish alarming links between food marketing and children's preferences, requests, consumption and obesity. It describes how advertisers target children who are too young to distinguish ads from truth and induce them to eat high-calorie, low-nutrient junk foods.[16] The report recommends that food companies voluntarily stop advertising unhealthy foods to children and, if they refuse, that Congress pass legislation prohibiting this. "Although marketers justify appeals to children as 'training' in consumer culture, as free speech, and as good for business, they are not selling just any consumer product: they are selling junk foods to children who would be better off not eating them," reads an editorial in the *New England Journal of Medicine*. "Companies succeed so well in this effort that business-as-usual cannot be allowed to continue."[17]

At least fifty countries already regulate television advertising to children. Australia bans food advertisements aimed at children younger than fourteen, Holland prohibits advertisements for candy to those under twelve and Sweden bans the use of cartoon characters to promote foods to children. The US merely regulates time allowed for commercials on children's shows: commercials may take up to twelve minutes per hour during weekdays but "only" ten and a half minutes per hour on weekends.[18]

It's time, as the report suggests, to ban such advertising to children. We might even want to consider regulations on advertising to adults, such as limiting the number of television advertisements per hour for unhealthy foods, and similar percentage limitations in other media as a start. More people object to controlling advertising for adults, as they're presumably able to make free choices. But just how free those are can be questioned, as Marion Nestle points out: "They [food companies] are putting $36 billion into directing those choices, and their methods are very effective."[19] Cigarette advertising was banned from television as part of a settlement with the tobacco industry. Hard-liquor advertising has been kept off the airwaves, with no notable adverse effect on the First Amendment.

Similarly, we make it illegal to sell children substances which adults are free to consume. Children and adolescents can't buy alcohol or cigarettes. Some parents allow teenagers to smoke or drink in their homes—but it's impossible to do so mindlessly without reflecting on why one is going against society's conventional wisdom about the unhealthiness of these substances. It might be well to begin to limit what can be sold to children—or put on children's menus in restaurants.

Prohibition

Everyone knows that Prohibition "failed." But failed at what? Failed to be popular? For sure—it was held in contempt by a good proportion of the populace. Failed to totally prevent drinking? Yes—it generated huge revenues for organized crime. But failed to *reduce* drinking? No. Failed to have any health impact? Again, no. Between 1906 and 1934, the annual per capita consumption of alcohol dropped from 9.8 liters to 3.7 liters as a result of Prohibition. This was followed by a decrease in liver-cirrhosis mortality. Deaths from cirrhosis fell from about sixteen per 100,000 population before Prohibition to eight per 100,000 population during Prohibition and for several decades after, as it takes fifteen to twenty years of heavy alcohol consumption before serious liver morbidity and mortality occur.[20]

Prohibition "failed" simply because the public wasn't in

favor of it. When I taught in Kuwait for a month after the first Gulf War, it seemed to me that their ban on alcohol worked well because most people supported it. Our laws prohibiting cocaine and heroin—and, for that matter, drugs like marijuana and hashish, which would never be outlawed in some parts of the world—also function well enough to reduce use, especially by minors, that we're willing to tolerate their increasing criminal revenue.

One country, the tiny Himalayan nation of Bhutan, has applied the prohibition solution to tobacco. In 2004, sales of tobacco products and public smoking became subject to fines of $210. Owners of shops and hotels violating the laws can lose their business licenses. Possession itself is not illegal, but there is a 100 percent tax on all tobacco products brought into the country for personal use.[21] "We want no pollution and good health for our citizens," Bhutanese Prime Minister Jigme Thinley stated in explaining the law.[22] Two years later, it seems to be well accepted, it has drastically reduced smoking in the country and the initiative has been praised by the WHO.

Remembering the research in Chapter 3 on how similarly refined foods and addictive drugs affect the brain, we should consider prohibiting some supernormal stimuli completely even for adults. Trans fats appear to be a deserving candidate. Unlike other supernormal stimuli, they don't appeal to us *more* than their natural counterparts. They taste as good as some saturated fats, store better than unsaturated oils and are much less healthy than either. There's nothing that can't be made without them.

Trans fats are still ubiquitous after years of adverse findings and efforts to eliminate them. In 2005, the Center for Science in the Public Interest had medical students buy two orders of French fries at the cafeterias of university teaching hospitals, children's hospitals and the three government agencies involved in dietary regulations. Fries from each facility were sent to a laboratory for analysis.[23]

Several hospitals' cafeterias served fries with an average of 4 to 6 grams of trans fats in six ounces—the range found in fast-food chains. So did one government agency; there were 5.8 grams of trans fat in the fries from the cafeteria at the USDA. Other hospital cafeterias had samples containing 2 grams or less of trans fats, which usually indicates that the fries were pre-fried in hydrogenated oil by the manufacturer and then deep-fried in nonhydrogenated oil at the cafeteria. Some hospitals seemed to think their fries were trans-fat-free because they hadn't accounted for the pre-frying by the manufacturer. Among the few that had no, or only trace amounts of trans fats were the cafeterias at the US Food and Drug Administration and the National Institutes of Health—further evidence that they're the ones whom we want overseeing our health.

Walter Willett, chairman of nutrition at the Harvard School of Public Health, commented: "Five to six grams of trans fat is a huge amount just from one serving. Food services usually use the same oils for cooking fish, chicken and other foods as they do fries, so if they've got the high level in fries, they've got it in lots of foods. People should be able to assume that hospitals are serving them the healthiest food possible," Willett says. "In this case, their trust has clearly been betrayed."

I'd say no one ordering strips of starchy potato deep-fried in any oil could "trust" they're being served "the healthiest food possible." Why do French fries belong on the menu in hospitals at all? Hospitals have finally banned smoking and no longer sell cigarettes.

The study got an immediate response from this select group of eating establishments. Several teaching hospitals and the USDA scrambled to produce press releases saying they were discontinuing trans fats immediately. None defended using them. Chain restaurants respond differently, however. The Center for Science in the Public Interest has been providing fast-food outlets with similar laboratory analyses for some time. They did recently force McDonald's to admit that their French fries contained one-third more trans fats than the chain's nutritional information listed.[24] When two similar consumer organizations filed class action lawsuits because McDonald's had publicized in 2002 that it was going to phase out trans fats by 2003, then failed to do so but didn't inform customers, McDonald's settled the lawsuits jointly for $8.5 million. Most of the money was earmarked to fund public service announcements about trans fats.[25] However, none of these actions have actually gotten the chains to remove trans fats. McDonald's says it's not as easy as they first thought—which is ludicrous: some of the hospitals did it virtually overnight.

New prohibitive laws might be an easier way to handle trans fats than these tenuous lawsuits. Denmark has banned oils containing more than 2 percent trans fat. Canada is setting up a regulatory commission to enact a similar ban.[26]

We already ban all kinds of things—we're not free to eat fish with the highest mercury counts. When there's disease contamination, fishing waters are closed even to private fishermen. We mandate smoke detectors in homes, there are regulations about electrical wiring and gas valves which bind not just contractors but those working on their own homes. Our laws don't consider it completely your business if you want to risk a house fire. You can't feed your children off lead-glazed plates. Older readers can probably remember when seatbelt law proposals were viewed as a major infringement on individual liberty. Recreational drug enthusiasts have been lobbying for legalization for decades without persuading the majority.

Balancing health and the collective good against the right to make individual choices is always a legitimate issue for debate. Answers lie not just in the degree of harm from a particular substance but also in how much the public views it as good or bad. Prohibiting fatty sweets or potato chips in the near future would spawn junk-food speakeasies and a Mafia trade in jelly donuts. But trans fats are not something to which people have formed emotional attachments. People would happily eat the same foods made with other fats. This is a good place to start, and a few local jurisdictions have—most notably New York City, which has a moderate proposal to phase out trans fats.

We need to see how many other negative eating patterns change through education and public awareness campaigns and whether other problem food components might become desirable—and possible—to actually ban. It is not coincidental that my suggestions in this chapter on societal reform are less specific than in the previous one on individual change. The personal path to health within our current environment is well-mapped if lightly trodden. Individuals have made the change—but an entire society never has. The original anti-tobacco activists didn't know how their first steps would evolve into others, how much would be achieved by education versus outright ban. If they had a specific game plan, it's a safe bet society followed it only roughly.

Some changes—even radical ones—will be voluntary. Others happen reluctantly to prevent harsher legislation—this is widely believed to be the case with vending-machine owners agreeing to cease stocking sugared sodas in schools. Food companies may decide there's as much money to be made off healthy products, especially with the right government incentives in place.

And—once in a while—there will be an act of idealism. Politicians from the farming belt rarely take on the USDA. Patrick Fitzgerald of the "fox and henhouse" criticisms was a Republican endorsed by George W. Bush in his first run for the Senate. Approaching a second term, with polls favoring him to win and any other Republican to lose, the Republican Party of his state wouldn't back him for the primary. Fitzgerald bowed out and Democrat Barack Obama easily won the seat. Fitzgerald didn't backtrack, apologize or even sound surprised through any of this; he gracefully exited back to a civilian career. Next, let's examine in more detail someone else who ignored self-interest to publicize important health matters.

Swimming in Ice Cream

John Robbins was born the heir apparent to the Baskin-Robbins Ice Cream Company which was founded by his father and his maternal uncle, Bert Baskin. Hugely successful, Baskin and the senior Robbins were personal friends of Richard Nixon. Young John swam in a backyard swimming pool shaped like an ice-cream cone and feasted from a home freezer packed with all thirty-two flavors. As an only child and only nephew, he was being groomed to run the business. Upon graduation from high school, however, John Robbins went to the University of California, Berkeley—in its revolutionary heyday. He recalls, "I began to have other questions besides, 'What flavor do I want?'"

After college, John fell out with his father, publicly renounced his inheritance and wrote a book, *Diet for a New America*.[27] It detailed conditions on farms where cattle are filled with antibiotics, hormones, appetite stimulants and pesticides—all of which are passed along to humans. Along with advocating vegetarianism, animal rights and a non-capitalist lifestyle, it devoted many pages to similar points about the consumption of animal milk as I covered in Chapter 3. Some of Robbins's observations include:

- Milk Producer's original ad campaign slogan: "Everyone needs milk." / What the Federal Trade Commission called the "Everyone needs milk" slogan: "False, misleading and deceptive."

- Milk Producer's revised campaign slogan: "Milk has something for everybody." / Increased risk of breast cancer for women who eat butter and cheese three or more times a week compared to women who eat these foods less than once a week: three times higher.

• The Dairy Council tells us: Milk is nature's most perfect food. / The Dairy Council doesn't tell us: Milk is nature's most perfect food for a baby calf, who has four stomachs, will double its weight in forty-seven days, and is destined to weigh 300 pounds within a year.[28]

When the book was published, Robbins's mother asked him, "Why did you write this book— just to hurt us?" A few years later, her brother, 240-pound co-owner Bert Baskin, died of a heart attack. John Robbins saw this as related to all the ice-cream, but his parents didn't. Robbins senior was also growing obese, and soon developed type-2 diabetes and high cholesterol. One day at his doctor's office, he was bemoaning the way his medications couldn't completely control either condition and the doctor told him there was only so much a pill could do. A diet was what he really needed and he would do well to read his son's book! Robbins's father took this advice, reconciled with his son and lost weight. The younger Robbins now says his father doesn't touch ice cream; the elder Robbins, who still runs the company, is mute on this point.

Whatever Oedipal interpretation one could read into this story, and despite reservations about the amounts of grain he wants us to eat, I find John Robbins an inspiring example of the change that is possible even within corporate America. If reconciling with his father results in a renunciation of the renunciation of the inheritance, perhaps we'll eventually have a huge major dessert chain feeding us nothing but pure fruit sorbets.

Battling Sloth and the One-Eyed Monster

Exercise and television habits deserve a similarly radical over-haul. As with eating, in these areas also we need to stop supporting detrimental activities, subsidize healthy ones and consider what we want to prohibit entirely.

Exercise for children already has a great model in the PE4life program. It's catching on in many school systems, but its basics—daily exercise involving noncompetitive fitness-building activities—should become national educational policy. We also need more playgrounds for preschoolers. It's a sad commentary when some neighborhoods' only jungle gyms are at their local McDonald's or Burger King.

Adults need a place to exercise even more than children, as it can't be built into the work day as easily as it can be required at school. Cities should build more bike paths and sidewalks, not more parking lots. Tolls on roads can be raised and public transportation—which always involves some walking—made

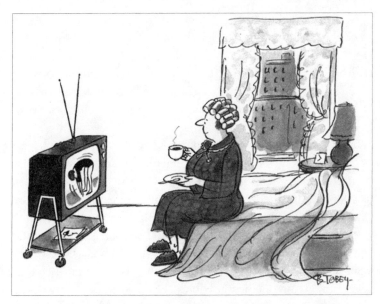

"Stand erect, feet twelve inches apart. Now bend forward to touch floor—keeping knees straight." (© *The New Yorker Collection 1974 Barney Tobey from cartoonbank.com*)

cheaper and pleasanter. Some medical plans already contribute to gym memberships as a preventive health measure. This is good, but we should go further, allowing lower premiums for those who exercise regularly—obviously at an appropriate level for an individual's condition. We already allow such rate incentives for non-smokers and non-drinkers.

We may need public service announcements containing snappy warnings such as RID's "Sedentary Death Syndrome" pronouncements. Or ones telling parents, "You may be worrying about protecting your child from the wrong thing. He/she has a .0006% chance of being killed by criminal violence if he/she plays outside and *fifteen times* that chance of dying of inactivity-related disorder if he/she doesn't."[29] Research shows not only that people rate these probabilities inaccurately, but that they just don't consider the latter at all.

We're not about to ban television in homes, but how about in public places? There are signs prohibiting cell phones in some bars, restaurants and doctors' waiting rooms where televisions still blast away. Remember the television researcher quoted in Chapter 5, who admitted that even he found himself staring up at public televisions in the midst of important conversations? It's a supernormal stimulus.

For young children, television should not be an acceptable part of daycare. Public service announcements should publicize its link to attention deficit disorder. But we probably need more than this, as television for the very young is actually increasing. Despite the American Academy of Pediatrics formally advising that no child under the age of two should be exposed to television at all, and that older children should see no more than two hours per day, this year two US advertising executives launched a round-the-clock television channel aimed at babies. To quote from their website: *"What age group should watch BabyFirstTV?* BabyFirstTV is an interactive tool for parents to engage their infants and toddlers ranging from six months to three years. Our content is specifically tailored to meet the needs of babies younger than three years and provides a safe, positive environment."[30]

BabyFirstTV has a page with testimonials from parents—most of which emphasize how long the child stays quiet and still while staring at the set. It's understandable why a tired parent might be tempted by this, but it's not a good sign in a wide-awake infant. However, BabyFirst assures parents that the positive effects are endorsed by "leading experts." The head of their own expert medical panel, Dr. Edward McCabe III of the Mattel Children's Hospital at UCLA, turns out to be in a department specializing in organ transplants and his own area of expertise is murine glycerol kinase deficiency. He's hardly a pediatric psychologist or psychiatrist. He and the rest of the panel make comments that sound unaware of the American Academy of Pediatrics' recommendation or the body of research on which it's based.

British critics are lobbying strongly against BabyFirst's plans to broadcast in England by 2007, dubbing it a "twenty-four-hour infomercial for attention deficit disorder" and "New Game for Baby: Shut Up and Watch." "Ten years ago," says David Burke, White Dot's British director, "the world was shocked to hear of infants tied to their chairs and ignored in a Chinese orphanage. Looking at the launch of BabyFirstTV, I wonder why we got so upset. Did they just need better-quality programs?"[31] In line with the American Academy of Pediatrics' recommendation, the US ought to backtrack and ban television aimed at children under the age of two.

Transcending Trans Fats: Worldwide and Long-Term Fixes

The solutions necessary and practical in the Third World differ from those for the US and other industrialized countries. Most people in the Third World still get vigorous exercise. Their food problems include scarcity—though the WHO recently announced that overfeeding is now a wider problem than starvation for the first time in history. And whether over- or underfed, both cultures are frequently under*nourished* because their food is largely made up of simple carbohydrates and saturated fats, short on vitamins. Poorer countries are not as permeated with fast foods. Certain categories, however, such as soft drinks, are even more of a problem. Babies and very young children sometimes get sugary sodas instead of milk for lack of education; when infant formulas are used, they're often mixed with water instead of milk—and contaminated water at that.

Obviously much of the world can't afford to spend the amount on food that the US or Europe or Japan can. Americans, if they choose, can buy vegetables grown anywhere in the world—more fully replicating the variety available to hunter-gatherers. If one has that selection, grains are not the best choice for the bulk of the diet. Ideally, whole grains should be a small fraction of what we eat. But in much of the Third World, whole grains supplemented with smaller amounts of vegetables and protein is the only practical, affordable alternative that's much better than what's eaten now. At its current population, the planet can't support a hunter-gatherer lifestyle or the sort of agriculture that fully replicates it. In the long term, lowering the birthrate to control population might solve many environmental issues, but this is obviously a many-generational solution.

Shorter-term, getting poor countries to stop refining grains is a priority. We must use this staple whole with its fiber, essential oils and vitamins intact instead of turning it into white flour, white rice, corn syrup and products manufactured from them. Whole grains need to be supplemented with some vegetables and protein sources—relying on those that are cheap and easy to grow locally. In Bangladesh, beans and pumpkins thrive readily and supply vitamin A and other nutrients. The UN's Food and Agriculture Organization—which is much more health-conscious than the USDA—has helped landless families develop gardens to grow these crops for at least three million people. In Thailand, the ivy gourd grows easily and is again a good source of vitamin A and some of the B vitamins. A project in the Jiangsu province of China initiated rice/aquaculture systems, which resulted in 10–15 percent increases in rice yields and, more importantly, 750 kilos of fish per hectare of rice paddy. The fish also help reduce the incidence of malaria by consuming mosquito larvae. In many more areas, soy is the cheapest producible healthy protein and can be a lifesaver.

Fortunately not everything modern agriculture has yielded is negative. Not all food has to be literally "natural." I don't believe we have to match the exact foods that our ancestors ate, but we ought to match their components. Humans demonstrably never ate seaweed or algae in the cradle of the human race, but when they later wandered close to oceans, they occasionally did. Now we can harvest much from the deep sea—even deep ocean fish is not exactly natural to our diet but is obviously nutritious. So are the less expensive and less depleted plants and microorganisms growing there.

Genetic engineering may also help us if we're careful with it. I'm not in agreement with foods boasting "non-genetically-engineered" in order to make a refined product of low nutritional value desirable. Obviously there's some danger of creating harmful new species and we do need regulations; that is beyond the scope of this book. But the risks are not so far beyond those of non-genetic agriculture: bringing crops from one continent to another has wiped out innumerable native plants, feeding herbivores leftover meat byproducts has brought us mad cow disease and breeding produce for appearance and sweetness has bred out nutrients.

Genetic engineering of crops has potential benefits—including the reversal of these centuries of ill-advised breeding. As James

Watson is fond of saying, "If scientists don't 'play God,' who will?" Golden rice is the most ambitious application of genetic engineering to date. This rice is produced by splicing three foreign genes—two from the daffodil and one from a bacterium—into japonica rice to provide vitamin A, which is deficient across much of Asia. All other current genetically-engineered crops are spliced with single genes, usually ones for resistance to disease. Golden rice has been criticized by environmentalists as a Trojan Horse, opening the developing countries to acceptance of genetically-engineered food. It has been pointed out that golden rice is not the silver bullet first perceived, because a standard serving currently provides only 10 percent of the US recommended daily allowance of vitamin A and only grows in temperate climates. But its inventors are advancing toward a tropical strain that supplies closer to 20–40 percent of daily requirements.[32] Even 10 percent of the RDA for vitamin A is sufficient to prevent blindness and death in children and adults, though it's not enough to prevent A-deficiency increases in childhood susceptibility to diarrhea, measles or a number of other infectious diseases.[33] Golden rice is a good model for slow, careful development: it originated with funding from the Rockefeller Foundation and is now backed by the World Health Organization.

Longer-term, science may find a way to re-engineer *us*. The current quests are for a pill that would make us less hungry or less prone to packing on fat cells. These would need to block or trick receptors. The problem with all existing diet drugs and any likely to be developed very soon is that our bodies' homeostatic mechanisms react to any foreign chemicals by readjusting, so that most new substances lose their effectiveness quickly. But it's possible that—as we come to understand the hormones involved in hunger, specific cravings and fat accumulation—we'll learn how to make ones so much like natural substances that they won't be subject to homeostasis. Medicine has achieved this with some medications, such as insulin and growth hormone. PYY, which signals fullness from the gut, leptin, which is released by fat cells when they sense high levels of lipids, or a substance that would block the hunger promoter ghrelin all might be candidates for such an approach.

Perhaps ultimately gene therapy—permanently going in and altering our programming—will be a solution, not just for those with unusually obesity-prone genotypes but for our average Paleolithic-designed selves. However, for people alive today and worrying about their own health or for government planners thinking about the current and next generations, gene therapy or even some perfected pill is not the immediate solution. We have to change food and exercise habits—and we have to change them radically, not moderately.

We really do treat animals better than ourselves—at least the ones we like: pets, zoo animals. There's a line of food for pets called Science Diet, and even a cat food named "hairball prevention." Human food names (any number of desserts have been dubbed "death by chocolate"), like the products inside, are designed to lure us into excess. This is more like the psychology of feed lots, in which cattle are coaxed to fatten themselves maximally just before slaughter, than like the way we treat animals for which we care.

The first step is to switch our mindset and stop believing that happiness can be had by unbridled indulgence of instincts. In a world increasingly designed to stimulate hunger continuously, this is a losing game. It's not anti-hedonistic to rein in, or redirect, instincts. Our pleasure system is robust and very flexible. Our brainpower can direct it—indeed, that's what it evolved to do. Scientific studies show that people experience similar levels of happiness long-term regardless of external events. Winning millions in a lottery or getting paralyzed in an accident—these make a modest difference for six months or less.[34] People in the most poverty-stricken countries are a couple of percentage points less happy than in the most affluent.[35] People who drink, don't drink, watch television, don't watch television, eat natural vegetables, eat junk food—all experience similar levels of life satisfaction. In fact, the only thing that makes a difference is chronic pain or consistent health crises—things our habits will produce.[36]

The pleasure mechanism can be shaped as to what it responds to; it doesn't have to be the other way around. We understand this more readily when we're thinking about the evanescent highs of drug addiction versus the pleasure of normal life interactions. But the same is true for diet and exercise habits. We can get used to deriving our set amount of pleasure from normal food and exercise patterns rather than supernormal ones. People get pleasure from what they have gotten used to getting pleasure from. Reward circuits in our brain will respond to the sugar in a handful of tart berries or from a whole cake, to the earned rest after exercise or the whole day on the couch, to real friends dropping by or the simulated laugh-track of a sitcom.

We need to get ourselves into a situation in which we get pleasure from activities for which our instincts were originally designed. This involves either people training themselves to ignore supernormal stimuli, to use their evolved brains to direct eating and exercise as discussed in Chapter 8—or to radically re-engineer our environment, as we've been examining in this chapter, so that it presents us with *normal* stimuli in normal quantities and frequency. When people heed the signs and don't feed the animals, the zoo denizens cease even thinking about marshmallows and chips and really do enjoy the greens. So will we.

Notes

1 Don't Feed the Animals

1. David Satcher, MD, US Sur. Gen., *The Surgeon General's Call to Action to Prevent and Decrease Overweight and Obesity*, Section 1.3: Economic Consequences and Section 1.2: Health Risks (Rockville, MD: US Department of Health and Human Services, 2001). See also D. B. Allison and others, "Annual Deaths Attributable to Obesity in the United States," *Journal of the American Medical Association* 282, no. 16 (October 27, 1999): 1530–8, for more detail on mortality estimates.
2. Gallup survey conducted November 3–5, 2003, news release, Gallup Organization, www.galluppoll.com/analyses.
3. Vending machine data from Nanci Hellmich, "School Vending Rated as Junk," *USA Today*, May 11, 2004, reporting a survey from the Center for Science in the Public Interest and data on the decrease in physical education programs.
4. Satcher, *Surgeon General's Call*, Section 1.3: Economic Consequences.
5. Alex Dominiguez, "Most Americans Will Be Fat Over the Long Haul: Nine Out of 10 Men and Seven Out of 10 Women Will Become Overweight," Associated Press, October 4, 2005, http://www.newsday.com /news/nationwide/wire.
6. "Social Trends Poll: Americans See Weight Problems Everywhere but in the Mirror," Pew Poll Report, April 11, 2006 http://www.pewtrusts.com /pdf/PRC_obesity_0406.pdf (accessed August 26, 2006).

7. Stephanie Nebehay, "U.S. Accused of Undermining World Obesity Fight," Reuters, January 16, 2005, http://today.reuters.com/news.

2 Which Came First: the Take-Out Fried Chicken or the Cholesterol-Laden Egg?

1. Dora L. Costa and Richard H. Steckel, "Long-Term Trends in Health, Welfare, and Economic Growth in the United States," NBER Historical Working Papers 0076 (National Bureau of Economic Research, Inc., 2005), www.nber.org, reprinted in Richard H. Steckel and Floyd Roderick, eds., *Health and Welfare during Industrialization* (Chicago: University of Chicago Press, 1997).
2. Marvin Harris, *Cannibals and Kings: The Origins of Cultures* (New York: Random House, 1977).
3. Richard Lee and Irven DeVore, eds., *Man the Hunter* (Chicago: Aldine, 1968); Marshall Sahlins, *Tribesmen* (Englewood Cliffs, NJ: Prentice-Hall, 1968); and Marshall Sahlins, *Stone Age Economics* (Chicago: Aldine, 1972).
4. Harris, *Cannibals and Kings*, 10.
5. Thomas Barfield, *The Dictionary of Anthropology* (Oxford: Blackwell, 1997), 202.
6. S. Boyd Eaton and Stanley B. Eaton III, "Hunter-Gatherers and Human Health," in R. Lee and R. Daly, eds., *The Cambridge Encyclopedia of Hunters and Gatherers* (Cambridge: Cambridge University Press, 1999), 451.
7. Peter Farb and George Armelagos, *Consuming Passions: The Anthropology of Eating* (Boston: Houghton Mifflin, 1980), 79.
8. Richard Lee, *The Dobe !Kung* (New York: Holt, Rinehart, and Winston, 1984), 36.
9. Lee and DeVore, op cit.
10. Jared Diamond, "The Worst Mistake in the History of the Human Race," *Discover* (May 1987), 64–6.
11. These figures are from Diamond, "Worst Mistake." Lifespans calculated from different fossil remains which result in slightly higher averages but similar decrements between hunter-gatherers and early farmers appear in J. Lawrence Angel "Paleoecology, Paleodemography and Health," in Steven Polgar, ed., *Population, Ecology and Social Evolution* (The Hague: Mouton, 1975), 167–90; Mark N. Cohen and G. J. Armelagos, *Paleopathology at the Origins of Agriculture* (New York: Academic Press, 1984); and Harris, *Cannibals and Kings*.

12. Mark Nathan Cohen, *Health and the Rise of Civilization* (New Haven: Yale University Press, 1989), 138.

13. Angel, "Paleoecology, Paleodemography and Health."

14. Harris, *Cannibals and Kings*, 14.

15. N.-G. Gejvall, *Westerhus: Medieval Population and Church in the Light of Skeletal Remains* (Lund: Hakan Ohlssons Boktryckeri, 1960).

16. Pia Bennike, *Paleopathology of Danish Skeletons* (Copenhagen: Almquist and Wiksell, 1985).

17. Evolutionary medicine experts believe that measles and smallpox most likely originated from related viruses in cattle, tuberculosis from a spirochete infecting cattle, pertussis from either pigs or dogs and both malaria and influenza from birds (with chickens and ducks probably infecting humans). For a discussion of the general issue of the evolution of human disease from illness in domesticated animals, see A. Cockburn, "Where Did Our Infectious Diseases Come From?," in Ciba Foundation symposium, *Health and Diseases in Tribal Societies* (Amsterdam: Elsevier, 1977), 103–13; P. Ewald, *Evolution of Infectious Disease* (New York: Oxford University Press, 1994) and G. C. Williams, "The Dawn of Darwinian Medicine," *Quarterly Review of Biology* 66 (1991):1–61. For more detail on the likely evolution of measles from the cattle disease rinderpest, see E. Norrby and others, "Is Rinderpest Virus the Archevirus of the Morbillivirus Genus?," *Intervirology* 23 (1985): 228–32.

18. A. Lucas and others, "Breast Milk and Subsequent Intelligence Quotient in Children Born Preterm," *Lancet* 339 (1992): 261–4.

19. A. Rode and R. J. Shepard, "Physiological Consequences of Acculturation: A Twenty-Year Study of Fitness in an Innuit Community," *European Journal of Applied Physiology* 69 (1994): 516–24.

20. Elena Boserup, "The Impact of Scarcity and Plenty on Development," in R. Rotberg and T. Rabb, eds., *Hunger and History* (Cambridge: Cambridge University Press, 1983), 185–209.

21. Mark Cohen, "The Significance of Long-Term Changes in the Human Diet and Food Economy," in Marvin Harris and Eric Ross, eds., *Food and Evolution* (Philadelphia: Temple University Press, 1987), 581.

22. Harris, *Cannibals and Kings*.

23. Eaton and Eaton, "Hunter-Gatherers and Human Health," 449.

3 Don't Be Too Refined

1. Richard Perez-Pena and Grant Glickson, "As Obesity Rises, Health Care Indignities Multiply," *New York Times*, November 29, 2003, A1.

2. Deborah Koons Garcia, *The Future of Food*, film (Mill Valley, CA: Lilly Films, 2005).

3. D. Dye, "Nutritional Value of Produce Has Declined over Half a Century," quoting *Journal of American College of Nutrition* (December 2004), Life Extension Foundation, http://www.lef.org/whatshot/2004_12.htm# nvop (accessed July 16, 2006).

4. "Origin of the European Cultivated Carrot and the Development of the Original European Carrot Material," M-105 (Wageningen, Holland: Institute of Horticultural Plant Breeding, June, 1957) and Farm Service Agency, US Department of Agriculture, http://www.fsa.usda.gov/ca/Kid_Pages/carrot_trivia.htm.

5. See Greg Critser, *Fatland* (Boston: Houghton Mifflin, 1993), 136–9, for a fuller discussion of the different metabolism of sucrose vs. fructose.

6. Kitty Keene, "Brave New World: Capturing the Flavor Bug from Microorganisms," *Food Processing*, March 1995.

7. Carlo Colantuoni and others, "Evidence That Intermittent, Excessive Sugar Intake Causes Endogenous Opioid Dependence," *Obesity Research* 10, no. 6 (2002): 478–88.

8. Diane Martindale, "Burgers on the Brain: Can You Really Get Addicted to Fast Food?," *New Scientist*, February 1, 2003.

9. J. Wang and others, "Overfeeding Rapidly Induces Leptin and Insulin Resistance," *Diabetes* 50 (2001): 2786–91.

10. A. Pocai and others, "Restoration of Hypothalamic Lipid Sensing Normalizes Energy and Glucose Homeostasis in Overfed Rats," *Journal of Clinical Investigation* 116 (2006): 1081–91.

11. Martindale, "Burgers on the Brain."

12. R. P. M. Mensink and M. B. Katan. "Effect of Dietary *Trans* Fatty Acids on High-Density and Low-Density Lipoprotein Cholesterol Levels in Healthy Subjects, *New England Journal of Medicine* 323 (1990): 439–45.

13. "*Trans* Fatty Acids and Coronary Heart Disease Risk," *American Journal of Clinical Nutrition* 62 (1995): 655S–70S.

14. W. C. Willett and A. Ascherio, "*Trans* Fatty Acids: Are the Effects Only Marginal?," *American Journal of Public Health* 84 (1994): 722–4.

15. Cathy Newman, "Why Are We So Fat?," *National Geographic*, August 2004, 46–61.

16. Gladys Block, *Journal of Food Chemistry and Analysis*, June 2004.

17. Reuters, "Researcher Links Obesity, Food Portions," December 18, 2003, http://today.reuters.com/news.

18. Brian Wansink, "Can Package Size Accelerate Usage Volume?," *Journal of Marketing* 60 (July 1996), 1–14.

19. Reuters, "Researcher Links Obesity, Food Portions."

20. Barbara Rolls, S. J. Kim and I. Fedoroff, "Effects of Drinking Water Sweetened with Sucrose or Aspartame on Hunger, Thirst and Food Intake," *Physiology of Behavior* 48 (1999): 19–26.

21. J. Yanovski and others, "A Prospective Study of Holiday Weight Gain," *New England Journal of Medicine* 342 (2000): 861–7.

22. Barry Popkin and others, "A New Proposed Guidance System for Beverage Consumption in the United States," *Journal of Clinical Nutrition* 83 (March 2006): 529–42.

23. S. P. Fowler, Abstract 1058-P, Proceedings of the 65th Annual Scientific Sessions, American Diabetes Association, San Diego, CA, June 10–14, 2005.

24. Daniel DeNoon, "Drink More Diet Soda, Gain More Weight," *Web MD*, June 15, 2005, http://www.webmd.com.

25. Lewis Carroll, *Alice in Wonderland* (London: Macmillan, 1865), 84.

26. Daniel DeNoon, "Drink More Diet Soda, Gain More Weight."

27. T. Davidson, "A Pavlovian Approach to the Problem of Obesity," *International Journal of Obesity* 28 (July 2004): 933–5.

28. Kim Painter, "A Gluttony of Glug-Glugging," *USA Today*, April 10, 2006, D6.

29. Justin Prichard, "Immigrants Outlive U.S.-Born Residents," Associated Press, May 26, 2005. http://www.newsday.com/news.

30. Ibid.

31. Nicholas Kristoff, "Dreams of Osama bin Laden," *New York Times*, October 12, 2004.

32. John Vidal, *McLibel* (London: New Press, 1997), 46–7.

33. Eric Schlosser, *Fast-Food Nation: The Dark Side of the All-American Meal* (Boston: Houghton Mifflin, 2001).

34. Bruce Upton, "Beyond Burgers," *Forbes*, November 1, 1999.

35. John Love, *McDonald's: Behind the Arches* (New York: Bantam, 1986).

36. B. Horovitz, "McDonald's Goes After the Small Fry," *USA Today*, October 8, 1998.

37. Jim Suhr, "Hardee's Monster Burger Creates Uproar," Associated Press, December 7, 2004, http://www.newsday.com/news.

38. Ibid.

39. Sid Kirchheimer, "Waistline-Friendly Fast-Food?," *Web MD*, November 17, 2003, http://www.webmd.com.

40. Sam Bradley and Betsey Spethmann, "The Key to Attracting Kids Is Toys, Toys, Toys," *Brandweek*, October 1994.

41. Jerry Pallotta, *The Hershey's Kisses Subtraction Book* (New York: Cartwheel Books, 2002). Amazon.com buying suggestions at http://www.amazon .com/Hersheys-Kisses-Subtraction-Book/dp/0439337798/sr=1-1/qid= 1157161008/ref=sr_1_1/103-4549742-6506231?ie=UTF8&s=books (accessed June 15, 2006).

42. Anne Underwood, "How to Flunk Lunch," *Newsweek*, September 16, 2002.

43. Janet Bingham, "Corporate Curricula: And Now a Word, Lesson, Lunch from a Sponsor," *Denver Post*, February 22, 1998.

44. Hellmich, "School Vending Rated as Junk."

45. Samantha Gross, "Nearly All Sodas Sales to Schools to End," Associated Press, May 3, 2006, http://www.newsday.com/news.

46. "Hamburger Joints Call Their Customers 'Heavy Users' but Not to their Faces," *Wall Street Journal*, January 12, 2000.

47. I found this quote in Vidal, *McLibel*, along with some details which do not appear to be accurate: e.g., Vidal describes the first Japanese McDonald's as opening near the blast site of Hiroshima when Fujita actually opened the first one in the Ginza shopping district of Tokyo. However, Vidal cites the quote itself to Love, *McDonald's: Behind the Arches*. This is indeed where this statement first appears in English; it is a highly positive book about McDonald's by a business journalist, written with the full cooperation of McDonald's management. Love documents numerous appearances of the statement in the Japanese press.

48. Den Fujita authored works titled *Make Money with Stocks the Jews Aim At* and *Jewish Trade Methods* (both Tokyo: Waninohon, 1972), and used phrases that get translated into English as "money-grabbing" when speaking of Jewish businessmen; however, Fujita claims he intended these stereotypes as high praise of what he saw as admirable economic acumen.

49. Sam Pollock, "China's Biggest Little Emperors Struggle to Tone Up," Japan Economics Newswire, August 8, 1999, http://www.japaneconomics .com.

50. Love, *McDonald's*, 435.

51. Vidal, *McLibel*, 42

52. "Where's the Beef? It's in Your Fries. For Hindis and Vegetarians, Surprise at McDonald's," *New York Times*, May 20, 2001.

53. Frank Sacks, "Study Raises Beef in Fast-Food Fry," *Chicago Tribune*, March 11, 1988.

4 Get a Move On

1. I first read about sea squirts in Daniel Dennett's *Consciousness Explained* (Boston: Little, Brown and Co., 1991). Dennett uses the animal that finds its home and then "eats its brain" for a different metaphor: "It's somewhat like getting tenure," he observes. For more detailed information on *Ciona intestinalis*, including research using its eggs, see Elizabeth Pennins: "Comparative Genomics: Truncate Genome Show a Little Backbone," *Science* 298, December 13, 2002, 2111–2.

2. 1980–2000 Dept of Transportation National Household Survey, http://www.dot.gov.

3. US Department of Health and Human Services, *Physical Activity and Health: A Report of the Surgeon General* (Atlanta, GA: Centers for Disease Control and Prevention, 1996).

4. Paul Williams, "Physical Fitness and Activity as Separate Heart Disease Risk Factors: A Meta-Analysis," *Medicine and Science in Sports and Exercise* 33 (2001): 754–61.

5. G. K. Zipf, *Human Behavior and the Principle of Least Effort* (Boston: Addison-Wesley, 1949).

6. News release from PRNewsWire accompanying David S. Kump and Frank W. Booth, PhD, "Sustained Rise in Triacylglycerol Synthesis and Increased Edididymal Fat Mass When Rats Cease Voluntary Wheel Running," *Journal of Applied Physiology*, April 19, 2005, 911–25, http://www.prnewswire.com.

7. S. Lees and F. Booth, "Sedentary Death Syndrome," *Canadian Journal of Applied Physiology* 29, no. 4 (August 2004): 447–60; discussion 444–6.

8. Noël C. Barengo and others, "Low Physical Activity as a Predictor for Total and Cardiovascular Disease Mortality in Middle-aged Men and Women in Finland," *European Heart Journal* 25, no. 24 (2004): 2204–11.

9. Christian K. Roberts and R. James Barnard, "Invited Review: Effects of Exercise and Diet on Chronic Disease," *Journal of Applied Physiology* 98 (2005): 3–30.

10. Lees and Booth, "Sedentary Death Syndrome."

11. Frank Booth and others, "Waging War on Modern Chronic Diseases: Primary Prevention Through Exercise Biology," *Journal of Applied Physiology* 88 (2000): 774–87.

12. News release from PRNewsWire accompanying Kump and Booth, "Sustained Rise."

13. Kump and Booth, "Sustained Rise."

14. Ibid.

15.News release from PRNewsWire accompanying Kump and Booth, "Sustained Rise."

16.John Ratey, *A User's Guide to the Brain: Perception, Attention, and the Four Theaters of the Brain* (New York: Vintage, 2002).

17.H. van Praag and others, "Running Enhances Neurogenesis, Learning, and Long-Term Potentiation in Mice," *Proceedings of the National Academy of Sciences* 96 (1999): 13427–31.

18.Carl Cotman, *Trends in Neurosciences* 25 (2002):295–301.

19.Van Praag and others, "Running Enhances Neurogenesis."

20.Donna DeFalco, "A Perfect Fit: District's Physical-Education Curriculum a National Benchmark," *Naperville Sun*, March 31, 2004.

21.D. Laurin and others, "Physical Activity and Risk of Cognitive Impairment and Dementia in Elderly Persons," *Archives of Neurology* 58 (2001): 498–504.

22.R. P. Friedland and others,"Patients with Alzheimer's Disease Have Reduced Activities in Midlife Compared with Healthy Control-Group Members," *Proceedings of the National Academy of Science USA* 98 (2001): 3440–5.

23.W. Stummer and others, "Reduced Mortality and Brain Damage after Locomotor Activity in Gerbil Forebrain Ischemia," *Stroke* 25 (1994): 1862–9, and E. Carro and others, "Circulating Insulin-Like Growth Factor I Mediates the Protective Effects of Physical Exercise Against Brain Insults of Different Etiology and Anatomy," *Journal of Neuroscience* 21 (2001): 5678–84.

24.K. R. Isaacs and others, "Exercise and the Brain: Angiogenesis in the Adult Rat Cerebellum after Vigorous Physical Activity and Motor Skill Learning," *Journal of Cerebral Blood Flow Metabolism* 12 (1992): 110–9.

25.W. P. Morgan and others, "Psychological Effect of Chronic Physical Activity," *Medical Science in Sports* 2 (1970): 213–7, established that general exercise improved depression scores in those who were clinically depressed. J. H. Griest and others, "Running as Treatment for Depression," *Comprehensive Psychiatry* 20 (1979): 41–54, found the same was true for running specifically.

26.D. Scully and others, "Physical Exercise and Psychological Well Being: A Critical Review," *British Journal of Sports Medicine* 32, no. 2 (1998): 111–20.

27.James A. Blumenthal and others, "The Effects of Exercise on Type-A Behavior," *Psychosomatic Medicine* 42 (1980): 289–96.

28.Scully and others, "Physical Exercise and Psychological Well-Being."

29. S. A. Paluska and T. L. Schwenk, "Physical Activity and Mental Health: Current Concepts," *Sports Medicine* 29, no. 3 (2000): 167–80; E. J. Doyne and others, "Running versus Weightlifting in the Treatment of Depression," *Journal of Consulting Clinical Psychology* 55, no. 5 (1987): 748–54; and E. W. Martinsen, A. Hoffart and O. Solberg, "Comparing Aerobic with Anaerobic Forms of Exercise in the Treatment of Clinical Depression," *Comprehensive Psychiatry* 30 (1989): 324–31.

30. M. Moore, "Endorphins and Exercise: A Puzzling Relationship," *Physician Sports Medicine* 10, no. 2 (1982): 111–4; R. R. Yeung, "The Acute Effects of Exercise on Mood State," *Journal of Psychosomatic Research* 2 (1996): 123–41; and D. Taylor and others, "Acidosis Stimulates Beta-Endorphin Release during Exercise," *Journal of Applied Physiology* 77 (1994): 1913–8.

31. C. Ransford, "A Role for Amines in the Antidepressant Effect of Exercise," *Medical Science in Sports* 14 (1982): 1–10.

32. "Is Suburban Living Making You Sick? Study Finds Sprawl Linked to Chronic Ailments," press release, *Public Health*, September 27, 2003.

33. Ibid.

34. Bradford McKee, "As Suburbs Grow, So Do Waistlines," *New York Times*, September 4, 2003.

35. Samatha Marshall, "Manhattanites Prove Pound-Wise," *Crain's New York Business*, April 19, 2004.

36. Ibid.

37. Katherine Seelye, "Cities Made for Walking May Be Fat Burners: Does Living in the Suburbs Make You Fat?," *New York Times*, June 20, 2003.

38. Graham Harvey, *The Forgiveness of Nature: The Story of Grass* (London: Jonathan Cape, 2001).

39. C. B. Field, "Sharing the Garden," *Science* 294 (December 21 2001): 2490–1.

40. Anemona Hartocollis, "Where You Live Can Hurt You," *New York Times*, February 27, 2005.

41. R. J. Ross and others, "Computed Tomography, EEG and Neurologic Examination in Boxers," and American Medical Association Council on Scientific Affairs, "Brain Injury in Boxing," *Journal of the American Medical Association* 249 (1983): 211–3 and 254–7. Two editorials in this issue called for a ban on boxing, and the British and Australian Medical Associations have since followed suit.

42. Anemona Hartocollis, "Where You Live."

43. DeFalco, "A Perfect Fit."

44. Patrick Perry, "Keeping Kids Fit for Life," *Saturday Evening Post*, July–August 2003.

45. DeFalco, "A Perfect Fit."

46. Charlotta C. Postlewaite, " 'New PE' Emphasizes Cardiovascular Fitness, Targets Healthy Heart Zone while Promoting 'Personal Best,' " *State News*, February 4, 2003.

47. Ibid.

48. Rosalind Rossi, "On Top of the World," *Chicago Sun Times*, April 5, 2001.

49. Perry, "Keeping Kids Fit for Life."

50. I. Dreyfus, "Full-Bodied Models Highlight Fitness Ads," Associated Press, January 5, 2004, http://www.newsday.com/news.

5 Thinking Outside the Box

1. Robert Kubey and Mihaly Csikszentmihalyi, "Television Addiction—How Easily We Are Harmed By Our Desires," *Scientific American*, January 25, 2002.

2. Ibid.

3. Robert Kubey and Mihaly Csikszentmihalyi, *Television and the Quality of Life: How Viewing Shapes Everyday Experience* (Mahwah, NJ: Lawrence Erlbaum Associates, 1990), cited a 1986 study by Byron Reeves of Stanford University and Esther Thorson of the University of Missouri.

4. Study by Robert Klesges of Memphis State University. cited in Kubey and Csikszentmihalyi, "Television Addiction."

5. Kubey and Csikszentmihalyi, "Television Addiction."

6. Darcy A. Thompson, MD, MPH, and Dimitri A. Christakis, "The Association Between Television Viewing and Irregular Sleep Schedules Among Children Less than 3 Years of Age," *Pediatrics* 116, no. 4 (October 2005): 851–6.

7. Lillian G. Katz, "Monitoring TV Time," *Parents*, January 1989.

8. John C. Wright and others, "The Relations of Early Television Viewing to School Readiness and Vocabulary of Children from Low-Income Families: The Early Window Project," *Child Development* 72 (October 2001): 1347–66.

9. Healy wrote as part of a commentary panel at the Children's Hospital and Regional Medical Center in Seattle, WA, in response to Dimitri A. Christakis, MD, and others, "Early Television Exposure and Subsequent Attentional Problems in Children," *Pediatrics* 113 (April 2004); http://www.seattlechildrens.org/ (accessed June 20, 2006).

10. UPenn Communications Dean George Gerbner, as quoted at http://www.ucgstp.org/lit/vt/vt03/tvfacts.htm.

11. Ibid.

12. K. Coon and others, "Relationships Between Use of Television During Meals and Children's Food Consumption Patterns," *Pediatrics* 101, no. 1 (January 2001): 167–76.

13. Johnnie Roberts, "TV's New Brand of Stars," *Newsweek*, November 22, 2004.

14. Correspondence between Sylvester Stallone and Bob Kovoloff dated April 28, 1983, was submitted to the Justice Department. It can be found at http://galen.library.ucsf.edu/tobacco/docs/html/2404.02/2404.02.1 .html.

15. Stuart Elliott, "Greatest Hits of Product Placement," *New York Times*, February 28, 2005.

16. Ibid.

17. Lorne Manly, "When the Ad Turns into the Story Line" *New York Times*, October 2, 2005.

18. Roberts, "TV's New Brand of Stars."

19. Ibid.

20. Greg Hernandez, "Product Placement Soars," *Los Angeles Daily News*, March 30, 2005.

21. Brooks Barnes, "Daytime TV Gets Generous with Plugs, *Wall Street Journal*, January 17, 2005.

22. The study, by the Advertising Research Foundation in 2005, was of 600 viewers, http://www.thearf.org.

23. Stuart Elliott, "More Products Get Roles in Shows," *New York Times*, March 29, 2005

24. Manly, "When the Ad Turns into the Story Line."

25. "International Federation of Competitive Eating," *Wikipedia*, http://en .wikipedia.org/wiki/IFOCE (accessed May 20, 2006).

26. Buck Wolf, "Competitive Eating May Be a Sport for the Thin," "The Buck Files," *ABC News*, "http://abcnews.go.com/Entertainment/Wolf Files/story?id=116496&page=1 (accessed May 20, 2006).

27. Mark Johnson, "Doctors Appalled by Societal Glorification of Binge Eating," Knight Ridder Newspapers, September 21, 2005, http://www .mercurynews.com.

28. Ibid.

29. Wolf, "Competitive Eating May Be a Sport for the Thin."

30. Johnson, "Doctors Appalled."

31. Barbara A. Dennison, MD, Tara A. Erb, MS, and Paul L. Jenkins, PhD, "Television Viewing and Television in Bedroom Associated With Overweight Risk Among Low-Income Preschool Children," *Pediatrics* 109, no. 6 (June 2002): 1028–35.

32. A. Grund and others, "Is TV Viewing an Index of Physical Activity and Fitness in Overweight and Normal-Weight Children?", *Public Health Nutrition* 4, no. 6 (2001): 1245–51.

33. Study by Dr. Frank Hu as reported at http://www.tvturnoff.org/facts&figs.

34. Frank Hu, MD, PhD, and others, "Television Watching and Other Sedentary Behaviors in Relation to Risk of Obesity and Type-2 Diabetes Mellitus in Women," *Journal of the American Medical Association* 289 (2003): 1785–91.

35. Thomas Robinson, cited at http://www.tvturnoff.org/facts&figs.

36. National Coalition on Television Violence, http://www.nctv.org.

37. American Psychological Association, http://www.apa.org.

38. "Monitoring TV Time."

39. R. Liebert and R. Baron, "Immediate Effects of Televised Violence on Children's Behavior," *Developmental Psychology* 4 (1972): 469–75.

40. Glenn T. Ellis and Francis Sekyra III, "The Effect of Aggressive Cartoons on Behavior of First Grade Children," *Journal of Psychology* 81 (1972): 37–43; O. Ivar Lovaas, "Effect of Exposure to Symbolic Aggression on Aggressive Behavior," *Child Development* 32 (1961): 37–44; Paul Mussen and Eldred Rutherford, "Effects of Aggressive Cartoons on Children's Aggressive Play," *Journal of Abnormal Social Psychology* 62 (1961): 461–4.

41. Katz, "Monitoring TV Time."

42. John P. Robinson and Jerald G. Bachman, "Television Viewing Habits and Aggression," in George A. Comstock and Eli A. Rubinstein, eds., *Television and Social Behavior: Television and Adolescent Aggressiveness*, A Publication of the Television and Social Behavior Program, Washington, D.C., U.S. Government Printing Office.

43. Charles K. Atkin and others, "Selective Exposure to Televised Violence," *Journal of Broadcasting* 23 (1979): 5–13.

44. David P. Phillips, "The Impact of Mass Media Violence on US Homicides," *American Sociology Review* 48 (1983): 560–8.

45. Brandon S. Centerwall, "Television and Violence: The Scale of the Problem and Where to Go from Here," *Journal of the American Medical Association* 267 (1992): 3059–63.

46. A. J. Romero and others, "Are Perceived Neighborhood Hazards a Barrier to Physical Activity in Children?," *Archives of Pediatrics and Adolescent Medicine* 155 (2001): 529.

47. Though these professional groups have rivalries that result in little clear consensus, on this matter they did agree. Other signatories to the recom-

mendations to Congress were the American Academy of Child and Adolescent Psychiatry, the American Psychiatric Association and the American Academy of Family Physicians.

48. George Gerbner, "The Importance of Being Critical: In One's Own Fashion," *Journal of Communication* 33 (1983): 20–3.

49. Gerbner, http://www.usgstp.org/lit/vt/vt03/tvfacts.htm.

50. Ibid.

51. White Dot, http://www.whitedot.org/issue/iss_front.asp (accessed June
18, 2006).

52. Reuters, "Want to Sex Up Your Love Life? Turn Off the TV," January 18,
2006, http://www.reuters.com/news.

53. Laura Berman, "A Kiss Is Lots More than a Kiss, Study Shows," *Chicago
Sun Times*, February 13, 2006.

54. http://www.tvbgone.com/cfe_tvbg_main.php.

55. TV Turnoff Network, "TV Facts and Figures: Quotes," quoting Drew
Henderson, http://www.tvturnoff.org/quotes.htm (accessed January 20,
2006).

56. Robert Welch, "Making Your Family #1," *Focus on the Family Magazine*,
January 1987, 4, reporting on a Michigan State University study.

6 You Can't Be Too Rich or Too Thin

1. Susie Orbach, *Fat Is a Feminist Issue* (London: BBS Publishing Corporation, 1997).

2. All official "Miss America" winner statistics, along with averages for
every age group, decade, etc., are posted at http://www.timestocome.com/
blogs/fat.html (accessed May 1, 2006). A few of the main statistics based
on those numbers are:

Decade	Average Age	Average Height	Average BMI
1920s	17.33	64.92"	21.01
1930s	18.42	66.17"	19.3
1940s	19.2	67.15"	19.47
1950s	19.97	66.97"	19.47
1960s	19.5	66.5"	19.24
1970s	21.4	67.15"	18.33
1980s	21.6	67.1"	18.26
1990s	22.4	68.8"	18.93
2000s	23	65'	20.3

3. D. Symons, *The Evolution of Human Sexuality* (New York: Oxford University Press, 1981).

4. Search done on May 10, 2005, yielded fifteen listings of mannequins for sale:

Date	Height	Chest	Waist	Hips
new	5'8"	34"	26"	34"
new	5'8"	[not given]	25.5"	34"
new	5'10"	33"	23"	34"
new	5'8"	32"	23"	32"
new	5'9"	32"	23"	33"
new	5'4"	34"	24"	34"
new	5'7"	33"	24"	30"
new	5'11"	31"	23"	32"
new	5'11"	31"	26"	33"
new	6'	33"	24.5"	35"
new	5'11"	31"	23"	32"
new	6'	32"	25"	32"
1980s	5'7"	31"	24"	30"
1980s	5'10"	32"	24"	30"
1980s	5'7"	31"	24"	30"
2004 Average	5'9.25"	32.23"	24.67"	32.42"
1980s Average	5'8"	31.33"	24"	30"

5. Alison Maxwell, "Beauty's Staying Power," *USA Today*, October 25, 2005.

6. C. Witcombe, "Women in Prehistory: The Venus of Willendorf," in *Images of Women in Ancient Art*, http://www.arthistory.sbc.edu/imageswomen/ (accessed May 1, 2006).

7. "The figurines must be viewed in the symbolic context of cave art, which is fundamentally religious": in André Leroi-Gourhan, *The Art of Prehistoric Man in Western Europe* (London: Thames and Hudson, 1968); "It is safe to reject any belief that they have religious significance": Charles Seltman quoted in Akira Kato, "The Paleolithic Venuses: Who are They? What are They?," http://free.hostdepartment.com/b/barclay1720/hist/paleo/venus.htm (accessed May 1, 2006).

8. See Witcombe, "Women in Prehistory," for more detail on these speculations.

9. Marcia-Anne Dobres, "Venus Figurines," in Brian M. Fagan, ed., *The Oxford Companion to Archaeology* (Oxford: Oxford University Press,

1996), 740–1; and Peter J. Ucko, "The Interpretation of Prehistoric Anthropomorphic Figurines," *Journal of the Royal Anthropological Institute of Great Britain and Ireland* 92 (1962): 38–54.

10. J. L. Watkins, *The 100 Greatest Advertisements 1852–1958* (New York: Dover, 1959), 66.

11. J. McLester, "Overweight and Public Health," *Journal of the American Medical Association* 82 (1924): 2103.

12. In R. Keyes, *Nice Guys Finish Seventh: False Phrases, Spurious Sayings, and Familiar Misquotations* (New York: HarperCollins, 1993), 5–20.

13. L. Rosenfeld and others, "Preferences for Body Type and Body Characteristics Associated with Attractive and Unattractive Bodies: Jackson and McGill Revisited," *Perceptual and Motor Skills* 89 (1999): 459–70.

14. M. B. Harris, I. C. Walters and S. Waschull, "Gender and Ethnic Differences in Obesity-Related Behaviors and Attitudes in a College Sample," *Journal of Applied Social Psychology* 21 (1991): 1545–77; C. E. Rucker III and T. F. Cash, "Body Images, Body Size Perceptions, and Eating Behaviors among African-Americans and White College Women," *International Journal of Eating Disorders* 12 (1992): 291–9; Jack Mearest, "Body Image: Gender, Ethnic, and Age Differences," *Journal of Social Psychology* 140, no. 4 (August 2000): 465; and "Body Size Preferences across Ethnic Groups," paper presented at the annual meeting of the North American Association for the Study of Obesity, 2000, quoted in Critser *Fatland*, 120.

15. P. Brink, "The Fattening Room among the Annang of Nigeria," in N. J. Pollock and I. de Garine, eds., *Social Aspects of Obesity* (New York: Gordon and Breach, 1995).

16. Ann M. Simmons, "Where Fat Is a Mark of Beauty," *Los Angeles Times*, September 30, 1998.

17. I. de Garine, "Sociocultural Aspects of the Fattening among the Massa," in Pollock and de Garine, eds., *Social Aspects of Obesity*.

18. Symons, *The Evolution of Human Sexuality*, documents these as the major components of female aesthetics across a broad array of human cultures.

19. Anonymous, http://www.timestocome.com/blogs/fat.html (accessed May 1, 2006).

7 The Bearable Lightness of Being: Medical Views on Ideal Weight

1. Hippocrates, *Aphorisms*, trans. Francis Adams, 2:44, http://www.classics mit.edu/Hippocrates.

2. Celsus of Alexandria, *De Medicina*, trans. W. G. Spencer (Cambridge, MA: Harvard University Press, 1935), 1:97.

3. Cecil Webb-Johnson, *Why Be Fat?* (London: Mills and Boon, 1923), 27.

4. Jean Frasmusan, *The Cure of Obesity*, trans. Elaine Wood (London: John Bale, Sons, and Davidson, 1930), 30–1.

5. Benjamin Franklin, *Poor Richard's Almanac*, 1733.

6. "Successful Treatment of Obesity in Tenth Century Spain," *Lancet* 346 (1995): 452.

7. Galen, *De Sanit Tuenda*, cited in Paulus Aegineta, *The Seven Books of Paulus Aegineta*, trans. Francis Adams (London: Sydenham Society, 1844), 1:8.

8. Paulus Aegineta, *The Seven Books*.

9. "Regimen Sanitas Salernanum" (Salernian Regimen of Health), quoted in Sander Gilman, *Fat Boys: A Slim Book* (Lincoln, Nebraska: University of Nebraska Press, 2004).

10. Maimonides, *The Book of Knowledge*, http://www.jewishhealing.com/diet-rambam.html (accessed May 5, 2006).

11. William Banting, *Letter on Corpulence Addressed to the Public*, 2nd ed. (London: Harrison, 1863).

12. William Wadd, *Comments on Corpulency* (London: John Ebers, 1829); and Cecil Webb-Johnson, *Why Be Fat?*

13. S. Weir Mitchell, *Fat and Blood and How to Make Them* (Philadephia: Lippincott, 1877), 15.

14. James Salisbury, *The Relation of Alimentation and Disease.* (New York: J. H. Vail and Co., 1888).

15. Titus 1:12 (New International Version).

16. Philistines 3:5 (New International Version).

17. Saint Thumaturgus Gregory a.k.a. Pope Gregory the Great, "Moralia in Job," trans. Michael Slasser, in *Fathers of the Church: Life and Works*, vol 98 (Washington, DC: Catholic University of America Press, 1998).

18. John D. Sinclair, introduction to Dante, *The Divine Comedy* (Garden City: Doubleday, 1959).

19. Patricia Harris, David Lyon and Sue McLaughlin, *The Meaning of Food* (Guilford, CT: Globe Pequot Press, 2005), 34.

20. Proverbs 23:21 (New International Version).

21. Proverbs 23:2 (New International Version).

22. Saint Thumaturgus Gregory, "Moralia in Job."

23. Jim Holt, "The Deadliest Sin: As Americans Prepare to Stuff Themselves with Turkey and Pumpkin Pie, Two New Books Ask What's So Bad about Gluttony, Anyway?," *Boston Globe*, November 23, 2003.

24. Kenneth Ferraro, "Firm Believers: Religion, Body Weight and Well-Being," *Review of Religious Research*, March 1998.
25. D. R. Bassett, P. L. Schneider and G. E. Huntington, "Physical Activity in an Old Order Amish Community," *Medicine and Science in Sports and Exercise* 36, no. 8 (August 2004): 1447; Gary E. Fraser, "Associations between Diet and Cancer, Ischemic Heart Disease and All-Cause Mortality in Non-Hispanic White California Seventh-day Adventists," *American Journal of Clinical Nutrition* 70, no. 3 (September 1999): 532S–538S.

Met Life Wrist Circumferences

FRAME SIZE	WOMEN			MEN
	Height: under 5'2"	*5'2"–5'5"*	*over 5'5"*	*over 5'5"*
Small	$<5\frac{1}{2}''$	$<6''$	$<6\frac{1}{4}''$	$5\frac{1}{2}''-6\frac{1}{2}''$
Medium	$5\frac{1}{2}''-5\frac{3}{4}''$	$6''-6\frac{1}{4}''$	$6\frac{1}{4}''-6\frac{1}{2}''$	$6\frac{1}{2}''-7\frac{1}{2}''$
Large	$>5\frac{3}{4}''$	$>6\frac{1}{4}''$	$>6\frac{1}{2}''$	$>7\frac{1}{2}''$

Later, Met Life developed elbow measurement to estimate frame size. Instructions were, "Bend forearm upward at a 90-degree angle. Keep fingers straight and turn the inside of your wrist toward your body. Place thumb and index finger of other hand on the two prominent bones on either side of the elbow. Measure space between your fingers on a ruler. (A physician would use a caliper.) Compare with tables below listing elbow measurements for *medium-framed* men and women. Measurements lower than those listed indicate small frame. Higher measurements indicate large frame."

Elbow Measurements for Medium Frame

MEN		WOMEN	
Height in 1" heels	*Elbow Breadth*	*Height in 1" heels*	*Elbow Breadth*
5'2"–5'3"	$2\frac{1}{2}''-2\frac{7}{8}$	4'10"–4'11"	$2\frac{1}{4}''-2\frac{1}{2}''$
5'4"–5'7"	$2\frac{5}{8}''-2\frac{7}{8}''$	5'0"–5'3"	$2\frac{1}{4}''-2\frac{1}{2}''$
5'8"–5'11"	$2\frac{3}{4}''-3''$	5'4"–5'7"	$2\frac{3}{8}''-2\frac{5}{8}''$
6'0"–6'3"	$2\frac{3}{4}''-3\frac{1}{8}''$	5'8"–5'11"	$2\frac{3}{8}''-2\frac{5}{8}''$
6'4"	$2\frac{7}{8}''-3\frac{1}{4}''$	6'0"	$2\frac{1}{2}''-2\frac{3}{4}''$

27. J. E. Manson and others, "Body Weight and Mortality among Women," *New England Journal of Medicine* 333, no. 11 (September 14, 1995): 677–85.

28. A. E. Field and others, "Impact of Overweight on the Risk of Developing Common Chronic Diseases during a 10-Year Period," *Archives of Internal Medicine* 161, no. 13 (July 9, 2001): 1581–6.

29. G. G. Rhoads and A. Kagan, "The Relation of Coronary Disease, Stroke, and Mortality to Weight in Youth and in Middle Age," *Lancet* 8323 (March 1, 1983): 492–5.

30. UNC News Services, press release no. 340, June 13, 2002, accompanying the publication of Mark Daniel, in *Diabetes Research and Clinical Practice* (June 2002), http://www.unc.edu/news/archives/jun02/danielo61102 .htm (accessed May 6, 2006).

31. E. Ravussin and others, "Effects of a Traditional Lifestyle on Obesity in Pima Indians," *Diabetes Care* 17, no. 14 (1994): 1067–74.

32. F. Booth and others, "Exercise and Gene Expression," *Journal of Physiology* 543, no. 2 (2002): 399–411.

33. Ibid.

34. Randy Schellenberg, http://randyschellenberg.tripod.com/anorexia truthinfo/id12.html (accessed October 6, 2006).

35. C. D. Lee, S. N. Blair and A. S. Jackson, "Cardiorespiratory Fitness, Body Composition, and All-Cause and Cardiovascular Disease Mortality in Men," *American Journal of Clinical Nutrition* 69, no. 3 (1999): 373–80.

36. K. Rexrode and others, "Abdominal Adiposity and Coronary Heart Disease in Women," *Journal of the American Medical Association* 280 (1998): 1843–8.

37. Amercian averages from Covert Bailey, *The Ultimate Fit or Fat.* (Boston: Houghton Mifflin, 1999). Hunter-gatherers' from Eaton and Eaton, "Hunter-gatherers and Human Health."

38. Obesity and the Risk of MI in 27,000 Participants from 52 Countries," Salim Yusuf and others, *Lancet* 366 (November 5, 2005): 1640–9.

39. "Want to Test How Healthy You Really Are?", *Daily Mail*, October 14, 2004. A study from Sweden published in January 2003 in the *International Journal of Cancer* found that your body fat percentage has a higher association with your risk of breast cancer than your BMI does.

40. F. Rous, "The Influence of Diet on Transplant and Spontaneous Tumors," *Journal of Experimental Medicine* 20 (1914): 433–51.

41. T. B. Osborne, L. B. Mendel and E. R. Ferry, "The Effect of Retardation of Growth upon the Breeding Period and Duration of Life in Rats," *Science* 45 (1917): 294–5.

42. C. M. McCay, W. E. Dilly and M. F. Crowell, "Growth Rates of Brook Trout Reared upon Purified Rations, upon Skim Milk Diets, and upon Combinations of Cereal Grains," *Journal of Nutrition* 1 (1929): 233–46;

C. M. McCay, M. F. Crowell and L. A. Maynard, "The Effect of Retarded Growth upon the Length of Life and upon the Ultimate Body Size," *Journal of Nutrition* 10 (1935): 63–79; C. M. McCay and others, "Retarded Growth, Lifespan, Ultimate Body Size, and Age Changes in the Albino Rat after Feeding Diets Restricted in Calories," *Journal of Nutrition* 18 (1937): 1–13; M. A. Rudzinska, "The Influence of the Amount of Food on the Reproduction Rate and Longevity of a Suctorian (*Tokophrya infusionum*)," *Science* 113 (1951): 11–12; and D. J. Clancy and others, "Dietary Restriction in Long-Lived Dwarf Flies," *Science* 296 (2002): 319.

43. D. F. Lawler and others, "Influence of Lifetime Food Restriction on Causes, Time, and Predictors of Death in Dogs," *Journal of the American Veterinary Medical Association* 226, no. 2 (2005): 225–31.

44. M. Gerbasse-Delima, M. Liu, R. Cheney, R. Mickey and R. Walford, "Immune Function and Survival in Long-Lived Mouse Strain Subjected to Undernutrition," *Gerontologia* 21 (1975): 184–93; and R. L. Walford and S. R. Spindler, "The Response to Caloric Restriction in Mammals Shows Features Also Common to Hibernation: A Cross-Adaptation Hypothesis," *Journals of Gerontology Series A: Biological Sciences and Medical Sciences* 52 (1997): 179–83.

45. Aspects of these findings appear in both J. Dhahbi, H. Kim, P. Mote, R. Beaver and S. Spindler, "Temporal Linkage between the Phenotypic and Genomic Responses to Caloric Restriction," *Proceedings of the National Academy of the Sciences* 101, no. 15 (2004): 5524–9, and in S. Cao and others, "Genomic Profiling of Short- and Long-Term Caloric Restriction Effects in the Liver of Aging Mice," *Proceedings of the National Academy of the Sciences* 98, no. 19 (2001): 10630–5.

46. N. Bodkin and others, "Mortality and Morbidity in Laboratory-maintained Rhesus Monkeys and Effects of Long-term Dietary Restriction," *Journals of Gerontology Series A: Biological Sciences and Medical Sciences* 58 (2003): B212–9; M. Lane and others, "Calorie Restriction in Primates," *Annals of the New York Academy of Sciences* 936 (2001): 287; and J. A. Mattison and others, "Calorie Restriction in Rhesus Monkeys," *Experimental Gerontology* 38, nos. 1–2 (January–February 2003): 35–46.

47. Robert Arking, "Aging: A Biological Perspective," *American Scientist* 91, no. 6 (November–December 2003): 508.

48. R. L. Walford, S. B. Harris and M. W. Gunion, "The Calorically Restricted Low-Fat Nutrient-Rich Diet in Biosphere-2 Significantly Lowers Blood Glucose, Total Leukocyte Count, Cholesterol, and Blood Pressure in Humans," *Proceedings of the National Academy of the Sciences* 89 (1992): 11533–7.

49. L. Heilbronn and others, "Effect of 6-Month Calorie Restriction on Bio-markers of Longevity, Metabolic Adaptation, and Oxidative Stress in Overweight Individuals: A Randomized Controlled Trial," *Journal of the American Medical Association* 295 (2006): 1539–48.

50. Roy L. Walford, *The 120 Year Diet* (New York: Pocket Books, 1991), revised and republished as *Beyond the 120 Year Diet: How to Double Your Vital Years* (New York: Four Walls Eight Windows, 2000). A more recent book by CR Society president Brian M. Delaney and Roy Walford's daughter, Lisa Walford, is *The Longevity Diet: Discover Calorie Restriction* (New York: Marlowe & Co., 2005).

51. The Calorie Restriction Society maintains an extensive website at http://www.calorierestriction.org.

52. L. Fontana and others, "Long-Term Calorie Restriction is Highly Effective in Reducing the Risk for Atherosclerosis in Humans," *Proceedings of the National Academy of Science* 101, no. 17 (April 27, 2004): 6659–63.

53. Luigi Fontana, presentation at the Calorie Restriction Society's annual meeting, Tucson, AZ, April 5–9, 2006.

54. B. Wilcox and others, "How Much Should We Eat? The Association Between Energy Intake and Mortality in a 36-Year Follow-Up Study of Japanese-American Men," *Journal of Gerontology: Biological Sciences* 59 (2004): 789–95.

8 Marching to a Different Drummer: Strategies for the Individual in an Unhealthy Society

1. Loren Cordain, *The Paleo Diet: Lose Weight and Get Healthy by Eating the Food You Were Designed to Eat* (New York: Wiley, 2001); S. B. Eaton, M. Shostak and M. Konner, *The Paleolithic Prescription: A Program of Diet and Exercise and a Design for Living.* (New York: Harper & Row, 1988); Ray Audette and Troy Gilchrist, *Neanderthin: Eat Like a Caveman to Achieve a Lean, Strong, Healthy Body* (New York: St. Martin's Press, 1999).

2. Nicholas Perricone, *The Perricone Prescription: A Physician's 28-Day Program for Total Body and Face Rejuvenation* (New York: HarperCollins, 2004).

3. Heroin addicts in the US have life expectancies which are decades shorter than non-users, but the vast majority of those deaths are incurred by risks specific to illegal use: overdose, HIV, hepatitis and violence related to procuring drugs. In England, where heroin in reliable doses is given to registered addicts, those who don't have infections from previ-

ous street use and who don't continue to use additional street drugs have lifespans only a few years shorter than the general population and better than those in methadone maintenance programs. For discussion of recent findings on these issues, see: P. Dukes, G. Robinson and B. Robinson, "Mortality of Intravenous Drug Users: Attenders at the Wellington Drug Clinic," *Drug & Alcohol Review* 11 (1992): 197–201; M. Frischer and others, "Mortality among Injecting Drug Users: A Critical Reappraisal," *Journal of Epidemiology and Community Health* 47 (1993): 59–63; A. Ghodse and others, "Deaths of Drug Addicts in the UK, 1967–81," *British Medical Journal* 290 (1985): 425–8; J. McCarthy, "More People Die from Methadone Use than from Heroin Misuse," Letters, *British Medical Journal* 315 (September 6, 1997): 603; and J. Marks, "Deaths from Methadone and Heroin," *Lancet* 343 (April 16, 1994).

4. Martin Seligman, *What You Can Change and What You Can't: The Complete Guide to Successful Self-Improvement* (New York: Ballantine Books, 1995).

5. D. J. Safer, "Diet, Behavior Modification, and Exercise: A Review of Obesity Treatments from a Long-Term Perspective," *South Medical Journal* 84, no. 12 (December 1991): 1470–4; R. R. Wing, "Behavioral Approaches to the Treatment of Obesity," in G. Bray, F. Bouchard and P. James, eds., *Handbook of Obesity* (New York: Marcel Dekker, Inc., 1998), 855–73; and R. W. Jeffery and others, "Long-Term Maintenance of Weight Loss: Current Status," *Health Psychology* 19 (2000): 5–16.

6. F. M. Kramer and others, "Long-Term Follow-Up of Behavioral Treatment for Obesity: Patterns of Weight Regain among Men and Women," *International Journal of Obesity* 13, no. 2 (1989): 123–36.

7. G. Kelly, *A Theory of Personality: The Psychology of Personal Constructs* (New York: W. W. Norton, 1963), 52.

8. Angela Hynes, "Absolute Willpower in Just 3 Steps," *Shape*, March 2005, 148.

9. Megan Oaten, "Longitudinal Gains in Self-Control," poster presentation at the Society for Personality and Social Psychology conference, Austin, TX, January 2004.

10. Hynes, "Absolute Willpower."

11. See Robert Pear, "Obesity Surgery Often Leads to Complications, Study Says," *New York Times*, July 24, 2006, gives a summary of several adult studies. M. Lawson and others, "One-Year Outcomes of Roux-en-Y Gastric Bypass for Morbidly Obese Adolescents, *Journal of Pediatric Surgery* 41, no. 1 (January 2006): 137–43 discusses adolescents.

12. I. Kirsch, "Hypnotic Enhancement of Cognitive-Behavioral Weight Loss Treatments: Another Meta-Reanalysis," *Journal of Consulting and Clinical Psychology* 64 (1996): 517–19.

13. A. Black and others, "Measurements of Total Energy Expenditure Provide Insights into the Validity of Dietary Measurements of Energy Intake," *Journal of the American Dietetic Association* 93 (1993): 572–9; and S. Heymsfield, D. Matthews and S. Heshka, "Doubly Labeled Water Measures Energy Use," *Scientific Medicine* 1 (1994): 74–83.

14. Anna Mudeva, "Poor Diet as Bad for Health as Smoking, Study Says," Reuters, May 29, 2006, http://www.reuters.org/news.

15. Ibid.

16. G. Cochrane and J. Friesen, "Hypnotherapy in Weight Loss Treatment," *Journal of Consulting and Clinical Psychology* 54 (1986): 489–92; and J. Stradling and others, "Controlled Trial of Hypnotherapy for Weight Loss in Patients with Obstructive Sleep Apnea," *International Journal of Obesity and Related Metabolic Disorders* 22, no. 3 (March 1998): 278–81.

17. M. S. Andersen, "Hypnotizability as a Factor in the Hypnotic Treatment of Obesity," *International Journal of Clinical and Experimental Hypnosis* 33 (1985): 150–9.

18. M. Barabasz and D. Spiegel, "Hypnotizability and Weight Loss in Obese Subjects," *International Journal of Eating Disorders* 8 (1989): 335–41.

19. T. Kavanagh, R. J. Shepard, and H. Doney, "Hypnosis and Exercise—A Possible Combined Therapy Following Myocardial Infarction," *American Journal of Clinical Hypnosis* 16 (1974): 160–5; and T. Kavanagh and others, "Exercise and Hypnotherapy in the Rehabilitation of the Coronary Patient," *Archives of Physical Medicine and Rehabilitation* 51 (1970): 578–87.

20. D. N. Bolocofsky, D. Spinler and L. Coulthard-Morris, "Effectiveness of Hypnosis as an Adjunct to Behavioral Weight Management," *Journal of Clinical Psychology* 41 (1985): 35–40.

21. I. Kirsch, "Hypnotic Enhancement of Cognitive-Behavioral Weight Loss Treatments." A somewhat different meta-analysis of many of the same studies disagreed and maintained that hypnosis enhances cognitive-behavioral psychotherapy only slightly, if at all: D. B. Allison and M. S. Faith, "Hypnosis as an Adjunct to Cognitive-Behavioral Psychotherapy for Obesity: A Meta-Analytic Reappraisal," *Journal of Consulting and Clinical Psychology* 64 (1996): 513–16.

22. One type of person who is highly hypnotizable was described in S. C. Wilson and T. X. Barber, A. A. Sheikh (ed). "The Fantasy-Prone Personality: Implications for Understanding Imagery, Hypnosis, and Cre-

ativity," in *Imagery: Current Theory, Research, and Application* (New York: Wiley and Sons, 1983): 340–87. This was confirmed in more controlled studies: S. J. Lynn and J. W. Rhue, "The Fantasy-Prone Person: Hypnosis, Imagination, and Creativity," *Journal of Personal and Social Psychology* 51, no. 2 (August 1986):404–8. My own studies found that there is a smaller group of highly-hypnotizables characterized by a trauma history and dissociative experiences but that even these people show many similarities in vividness of imagery with "fantasizers": D. L. Barrett, "Fantasizers and Dissociaters: An Empirically-Based Schema of Two Types of Deep Trance Subjects," *Psychological Reports* 71 (1992): 1011–14; and D. L. Barrett, "Fantasizers and Dissociaters: Two Types of High Hypnotizables, Two Imagery Styles," in R. Kusendorf, N. Spanos and B. Wallace, eds., *Hypnosis and Imagination* (New York: Baywood, 1996): 123–35.

23. D. E. Thorne and others, "Are 'Fat-Girls' More Hypnotically Susceptible?", *Psychological Reports* 38 (1976): 267–70.

24. Karin Michels and Anders Ekbom, "Caloric Restriction and Incidence of Breast Cancer," *Journal of the American Medical Association* 291 (2004): 1226–30, reports a greater than 50 percent reduction for breast cancer risk for women who have been hospitalized before age forty with a diagnosis of anorexia nervosa. I. Mellemkjaer and others, "Anorexia Nervosa and Cancer Risk," *Cancer Causes Control* 12, no. 2 (February 2001): 173–7, report a reduced rate of total cancers for both genders.

25. The National Weight Control Registry is at http://www.nwcr.ws.

26. Statistics based on "An Interview with Rena Wing: The Fight Against Flab," *Nutrition Action Health Letter*, December 1997, 2, and on data at http://www.nwcr.ws (accessed June 1, 2006).

9 Changing the Drumbeat: Strategies for a Healthy Society

1. Carolyn Lochhead, "Fatuous Response to Obesity," *SF Gate*, September 2, 2002, http://www.sfgate.com/cgi-bin/article.cgi?file=/c/a/2002/09/02/ED139862.DTL&type=printable.

2. Center for Science in the Public Interest, "Help Kill the Cheeseburger Bill," http://www.cspinet.org/takeaction/index.html (accessed July 2, 2006).

3. Libby Quaid, "Bill Targets State Food Label Warnings," Associated Press, August 20, 2006, http://www.newsday.com/news.

4. "USDA Role In Food Pyramid Criticized," *Chicago Tribune*, October 14, 2003.

5. "Farm Commodity Programs: A Short Primer," Congressional Research Service Report, June 20, 2002.

6. Research Report, vol. LXXII, no. 22 (Great Barrington, MA: American Institute for Economic Research, 2005).

7. US Department of Agriculture, "Inspection and Grading," fact sheet, http://www.fsis.usda.gov/Fact_Sheets/Inspection_&_Grading/index.asp.

8. John Robbins, Diet for a New America (Walpole, NH: Stillpoint Publications, 1987).

9. Michael Sloan, "National Dietary Guidelines Rewritten to Favor Industry," from Greenwatch, http://www.moveon.org/ (accessed May 10, 2006).

10. "USDA Role In Food Pyramid Criticized."

11. Eric Morath, "Senator Can't Stomach U.S. Food Pyramid Guidelines," St. Louis Post-Dispatch, October 5, 2003.

12. "USDA Role In Food Pyramid Criticized."

13. M. Higgins, "Study Finds Deficiencies in the US," Washington Times, September 30, 2005.

14. R. D. Utiger, "Need for More Vitamin D," editorial in New England Journal of Medicine 338, no. 12 (March 19, 1998): 828–9.

15. Scott Hodge, "For Big Franchises, Money to Go: Is the SBA Dispensing Corporate Welfare?," Washington Post, November 30, 1997.

16. J. M. McGinnis, J. A. Gootman, and V. I. Kraak, eds. Food Marketing to Children and Youth: Threat or Opportunity? (Washington, DC: National Academies Press, 2006), summarized in Marion Nestle, "Food Marketing and Childhood Obesity—A Matter of Policy," New England Journal of Medicine 354, no. 24 (June 15, 2006): 2527–9.

17. Ibid.

18. Ibid.

19. Quoted in J. M. Hirsch, "Food Companies a Target in Obesity Fight," Associated Press, March 19, 2006, http://www.newsday.com/news.

20. A. Hetal and others, "Primary Prevention of Cirrhosis: Public Health Strategies That Can Make a Difference," Postgraduate Medicine 115, no. 1 (January 2004), www.postgradmed.com/issues/2004/01-04/kavsan.htm.

21. "Bhutan Forbids All Tobacco Sales," BBC News, December 17, 2004.

22. Suman Chakrabarti, "Bhutan Aims to Be First Country to Ban Tobacco," Inter Press Service, February 18, 2005, http://www.bhootan.org/modules.php?op=modload&name=News&file=article&sid=25&POSTNUKESID=6fe105c4acf7f9de96c954bocfb93817.

23. Nanci Hellmich, "You Really Don't Want Fries with That," USA Today, February 7, 2005.

24. Pallavi Gogoi, "McDonald's Breaks Out Nutritional Info on New Wrappers," *BusinessWeek*, February 18, 2006.

25. Associated Press, "Vegan Sues McDonald's Over French Fries," February 17, 2005, http://www.newsday.com/news. and Ban Trans Fats, "The Oreo Case," http://www.bantransfats.com/theoreocase.html (accessed August 3, 2006).

26. Ban Trans Fats, "The Oreo Case."

27. Robbins, *Diet for a New America*.

28. Linda Hardesty, "Dead Meat," *The Metropolitan* 20, no. 7.

29. Statistics from Centers for Disease Control, http://www.cdc.gov/nchs/fastats/homicide.htm, and Lees and Booth, "Sedentary Death Syndrome."

30. http://www.babyfirsttv.com/faq.asp#1.

31. http://www.whitedot.co.uk (accessed May 10, 2006).

32. P. Parameswaran, "Europe's 'golden' rice arrives in Asia amid controversy," Agence France-Presse, February 25, 2001, http://www.biotech-info.net/asian_controversy.html.

33. Golden Rice Project, "Biofortified Rice," http://www.goldenrice.org.

34. D. T. Gilbert and J. E. J. Ebert, "Decisions and Revisions: The Affective Forecasting of Changeable Outcomes," *Journal of Personality and Social Psychology* 82 (2002): 503–14; and T. D. Wilson, J. Meyers and D. T. Gilbert, "Lessons from the Past: Do People Learn from Experience That Emotional Reactions Are Short Lived?," *Personality and Social Psychology Bulletin* 27 (2001): 1648–61.

35. Ed Diener and Eunkook M. Suh, "National Differences in Subjective Well-Being," in D. Kahneman, E. Diener and N. Schwarz, eds., *Well-Being: The Foundations of Hedonic Psychology* (New York: Russell Sage Foundation, 1999), 434–50.

36. For a popular discussion of these results see Philip Hilts, "In Forecasting Their Emotions, Most People Flunk Out," *New York Times*, February 16, 1999. For more detail on research findings, see R. Veenhoven, World Database of Happiness, "Bibliography," http://www.worlddatabaseof happiness.eur.nl.

Acknowledgments

I want to thank all of my friends and colleagues who read and critiqued early drafts of this book. Morton Schatzman and David Spiegel provided everything from line edits to expertise as physicians. Don Symons supplemented my rudimentary knowledge of evolutionary anthropology. My friends Olga Michnikov and Ellie Tonkin read, reread and provided invaluable suggestions and support.

I'm grateful to the organizers of both writing groups to which I belong: Andrew Szanton, who can edit the most turgid academic sentences into perky prose, and Alyce Getler, who kept me focused on my evolutionary premise. And thanks to members of both groups for all their suggestions and encouragement: James Tobin, Judah Leblang, Ian Ruderman, Lisa Najavits, Beth Rider, Ayse Atasoyla, Patti Heyman and Ruth Cope. Friends and family who read parts of this book, commented and supported me through it include Barbara Barrett, Carol Oen, Roger Carlsmith, Alan Lightman, Will Lawrence, Ben Campbell, David Simpson and Vivian Schatzman. John Ratey lent his expertise to the exercise chapter. At Norton, my editor, Angela von der Lippe, and her assistant, Lydia Fitzpatrick, shepherded the book into print with tireless attention to detail.

I also wish to express my appreciation to the people who, over the years, have shared their expertise on these topics: Deborah Hulihan, Dan Brown and the rest of the staff at Cambridge Hospital's Behavioral Medicine Program, who taught me much about psychological interventions in health as I worked alongside them; Arreed Barabasz, with whom I co-lead hypnosis for weight and fitness workshops at national meetings; and the staff and members of Mike's Original Gym, who make regular exercise enjoyable.

INDEX

Page numbers in *italics* refer to illustrations.
Page numbers beginning with 215 refer to notes.